T0248759

SBAs, EMQs & SAQs in the SPECIALTIES

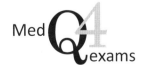

Matthew Hanks

tfm Publishing Limited, Castle Hill Barns, Harley, Shrewsbury, SY5 6LX, UK
Tel: +44 (0)1952 510061; Fax: +44 (0)1952 510192
E-mail: info@tfmpublishing.com; Web site: www.tfmpublishing.com

Editing, design & typesetting: Nikki Bramhill BSc Hons Dip Law
Cover photo: © iStock.com
Professional medical team (cyano66) — stock photo ID: 891531868

First edition: © 2021
Paperback   ISBN: 978-1-913755-00-3
E-book editions: © 2021
ePub   ISBN: 978-1-913755-01-0
Mobi   ISBN: 978-1-913755-02-7
Web pdf   ISBN: 978-1-913755-03-4

Printed by Gutenberg Press Ltd., Gudja Road, Tarxien, GXQ 2902, Malta
Tel: +356 2398 2201; Fax: +356 2398 2290
E-mail: info@gutenberg.com.mt; Web site: www.gutenberg.com.mt

Contents

About the Editor

Dr. Matthew Hanks graduated from the University of Sheffield in 2015 with an MBChB in medicine; prior to this Matthew studied for a BSc Biomedical Science degree in Sheffield graduating in 2010 with a first class honours degree. He has a keen interest in teaching and has devised many different teaching programmes for students which have been engaging and received positive feedback. He now hopes to take this passion further by providing students with resources that are both useful and informative to enhance their learning opportunities.

Contributors

Dr. Gemma Adams MBChB
Clinical Fellow in General Medicine and Geriatrics, South Yorkshire Deanery

Dr. Jack Baskerville BMedSci MBChB
Locum Senior House Officer, South Yorkshire Region

Dr. Rebecca Marlor BMedSci (Hons) MBChB
CT2 Core Medical Trainee, South Yorkshire Deanery

Dr. Katherine McPhail BMedSci MBChB
Clinical Fellow in Critical Care, Northern Deanery

Acknowledgements

I would like to thank all those who have taken the time to contribute to this title which is the amalgamation of knowledge from professionals studying and working all over the United Kingdom; without their hard work and dedication, this book would not have been possible.

I would like to thank Megan Ward and Glenda Hanks for their patience whilst the book has taken shape and the many nights of proofreading the text to ensure it will be useful for students. Koda and Joel Ward have provided a useful distraction when required!

Finally, the road to medical finals is a long one and this is the last major hurdle to becoming a doctor; the many hours of hard work and dedication already demonstrated in getting this far is about to pay off. All that is left to say is good luck!

Matthew Hanks
May 2020

Normal reference values

Please note normal reference values may vary between different hospitals.

Hb	Male 131-166g/L
	Female 110-147g/L
MCV	81-96fL
Platelets	150-400 x 10^9/L
WCC	3.5-9.5 x 10^9/L
Neutrophils	1.7-6.5 x 10^9/L
Lymphocytes	1.0-3.0 x 10^9/L
Eosinophils	0.04-0.5 x 10^9/L
Basophils	0.0-0.25 x 10^9/L
Sodium	133-146mmol/L
Potassium	3.5-5.3mmol/L
Urea	2.5-7.8mmol/L
Creatinine	62-106µmol/L
eGFR	>90
Calcium	2.25-2.5mmol/L
Total protein	60-80g/L
Globulin	18-36g/L
Bilirubin	0-21µmol/L
ALT	0-41iU/L
ALP	30-130iU/L

AST	0-35iU/L
Albumin	35-50g/L
PT	10.1-11.8 seconds
APTT	20.2-28.7 seconds
Thrombin time	11.3-17.4 seconds
Fibrinogen	2.0-4.0g/L
CRP	0-5mg/L

Abbreviations

ACTH	Adrenocorticotrophic hormone
ADHD	Attention deficit hyperactivity disorder
AF	Atrial fibrillation
AFP	Alpha fetoprotein
AKI	Acute kidney injury
ALL	Acute lymphoblastic leukaemia
ALP	Alkaline phosphatase
ALT	Alanine aminotransferase
AML	Acute myeloid leukaemia
ANA	Antinuclear antibodies
ANCA	Anti-neutrophil cytoplasmic antibodies
APTT	Activated partial thromboplastin time
ARMD	Age-related macular degeneration
ASD	Atrial septal defect
AST	Aspartate aminotransferase
AV	Atrioventricular
BAI	Beck Anxiety Inventory
BDI	Beck Depression Inventory
β-HCG	Beta human chorionic gonadotropin
BMI	Body Mass Index
CA	Cancer antigen
CABG	Coronary artery bypass grafting
CBT	Cognitive behavioural therapy
CEA	Carcinoembryonic antigen
CIN	Cervical intraepithelial neoplasia
CFTR	Cystic fibrosis transmembrane conductance regulator
CKD	Chronic kidney disease

COPD	Chronic obstructive pulmonary disease
CRP	C-reactive protein
CT	Computed tomography
DDH	Developmental dysplasia of the hip
DNA	Deoxyribose nucleic acid
DVT	Deep vein thrombosis
ECG	Electrocardiogram
ESR	Erythrocyte sedimentation rate
FBC	Full blood count
FIGO	International Federation of Gynaecology and Obstetrics
FSH	Follicle stimulating hormone
GFR	Glomerular filtration rate
GGT	Gamma-glutamyl transferase
GI	Gastrointestinal
GnRH	Gonadotropin-releasing hormone
GORD	Gastro-oesophageal reflux disease
GTN	Glyceryl trinitrate
HADS	Hospital Anxiety and Depression Scale
Hb	Haemoglobin
HELLP	Haemolysis (H), elevated liver enzymes (EL) and low platelet count (LP)
HIV	Human immunodeficiency virus
HPV	Human papilloma virus
HRT	Hormone replacement therapy
IM	Intramuscular
IQ	Intelligence quotient
IUD	Intrauterine device
IUGR	Intrauterine growth restriction
IUS	Intrauterine system
IV	Intravenous
LDH	Lactate dehydrogenase
LFT	Liver function test
LH	Luteinising hormone

LLETZ	Large loop excision of the transformation zone
MAOI	Monoamine oxidase inhibitor
MCV	Mean corpuscular volume
MDT	Multidisciplinary team
MEN	Multiple endocrine neoplasia
MHA	Mental Health Act
MRI	Magnetic resonance imaging
MS	Multiple sclerosis
MSUD	Maple syrup urine disease
NAPBQI	N-acetyl-p-benzoquinone imine
NICE	National Institute for Health and Care Excellence
NMS	Neuroleptic malignant syndrome
NPH	Normal pressure hydrocephalus
NSAID	Non-steroidal anti-inflammatory drug
NSPCC	National Society for the Prevention of Cruelty to Children
PAN	Polyarteritis nodosa
PAPP-A	Pregnancy-associated plasma protein-A
PCOS	Polycystic ovary syndrome
PEFR	Peak expiratory flow rate
PHQ-9	Patient Health Questionnaire 9
PID	Pelvic inflammatory disease
PKU	Phenylketonuria
PPH	Postpartum haemorrhage
PPI	Proton pump inhibitor
PSA	Prostate-specific antigen
PT	Prothrombin time
PTH	Parathyroid hormone
RAPD	Relative afferent pupillary defect
RAST	Radioallergosorbent test
RF	Rheumatoid factor
SARI	Serotonin antagonist and reuptake inhibitor
SIADH	Syndrome of inappropriate antidiuretic hormone secretion
SIRS	Systemic inflammatory response syndrome

SLE	Systemic lupus erythematosus
SNRI	Serotonin-norepinephrine reuptake inhibitor
SSRI	Selective serotonin reuptake inhibitor
STI	Sexually transmitted infection
SUDEP	Sudden unexpected death in epilepsy
TB	Tuberculosis
TCA	Tricyclic antidepressant
TENS	Transcutaneous electrical nerve stimulation
TFT	Thyroid function test
TIA	Transient ischaemic attack
TNM	Tumour, node, metastasis
TSH	Thyroid-stimulating hormone
TTG	Tissue transglutaminase
U&E	Urea & Electrolytes
USS	Ultrasound scan
UTI	Urinary tract infection
VBG	Venous blood gas
VEGF	Vascular endothelial growth factor
VSD	Ventricular septal defect
WCC	White cell count
WHO	World Health Organization

Section 1
Questions

Chapter 1

Dermatology
QUESTIONS

Single best answer questions

1) An 80-year-old nursing home resident complains of an intensely itchy rash. On examination, you find burrows between his finger webs. What first-line treatment would you offer him?

a. Topical emollients.
b. Permethrin cream.
c. Antihistamines.
d. Topical steroids.

2) A 24-year-old female developed a single oval plaque on her trunk 1 week ago which has now developed into multiple oval tawny lesions across the whole trunk, upper arms and legs. What is the most likely diagnosis?

a. Guttate psoriasis.
b. Pityriasis versicolor.
c. Lichen planus.
d. Pityriasis rosea.

3) A 15-year-old male presents to his primary care doctor with a new-onset rash. He is previously fit and well other than a sore throat 2 weeks ago which was treated with a course of antibiotics. On examination, there are multiple small drop-like salmon pink lesions present on his arms, legs and body. What is the most likely diagnosis?

a. Drug eruption.
b. Guttate psoriasis.
c. Lichen planus.
d. Eczema.

4) A concerned mother brings her 8-year-old son to the emergency department with a new-onset, palpable, non-blanching purpuric rash on his shins and buttocks over the last 2 days. He is also complaining of abdominal pain and has low-grade pyrexia at 37.8°C. What is the most likely diagnosis?

a. Meningococcal septicaemia.
b. Haemolytic uraemic syndrome.
c. Henoch-Schönlein purpura.
d. Psoriasis.

5) A 28-year-old Afro-Caribbean female presents to her primary care doctor with discrete, red tender nodules bilaterally on her shins and a dry cough. Given the most likely diagnosis what would you expect to find on her chest X-ray?

a. Hilar lymphadenopathy.
b. Bilateral consolidation.
c. Bilateral pleural effusions.
d. Cardiomegaly.

6) An 83-year-old life-long smoker with a chronic cough presents to his primary care doctor complaining of muscle weakness noting a particular difficulty when getting out of chairs. On examination, you notice a heliotrope rash across his face and back. What is the most likely diagnosis?

a. Polymyalgia rheumatica.
b. Osteoarthritis.
c. Dermatomyositis.
d. Polymyositis.

7) A 34-year-old female is admitted to the medical assessment unit feeling generally unwell with a painful leg. On examination, it is noted her lower left limb is hot, red, swollen and she is pyrexial; her blood tests show a raised white cell count and CRP. Given the most likely diagnosis, which of the following is the most appropriate initial management?

a. Venous Doppler.
b. Intravenous antibiotics.
c. Joint aspiration.
d. Conservative management.

8) A mother brings her 4-year-old daughter to her primary care doctor. She has been off her food with low-grade pyrexia for a couple of days and has now developed a rash. On examination, she doesn't look unwell; you notice vesicles on her palms, trunk and buccal mucosa. What is the most likely diagnosis?

a. Hand, foot and mouth disease.
b. Chickenpox.
c. Kawasaki disease.
d. Herpes simplex.

9) A 29-year-old female presents to her primary care doctor concerned about skin changes she has noticed. She is normally fit and well, has no drug allergies and takes levothyroxine daily. On examination, there are symmetrical patches of depigmented skin. What is the most likely diagnosis?

a. Eczema.
b. Lichen sclerosis.
c. Idiopathic hypomelanosis.
d. Vitiligo.

10) A 19-year-old hairdresser sees her primary care doctor with redness, itching and pain in her hands which she finds is worse following a day at work. You suspect occupational contact dermatitis. What kind of hypersensitivity reaction is this an example of?

a. Type I hypersensitivity reaction.
b. Type II hypersensitivity reaction.
c. Type III hypersensitivity reaction.
d. Type IV hypersensitivity reaction.

11) A 4-year-old is taken to the primary care doctor by his mother. He has a background of atopic eczema and has developed a golden crusting over the eczematous lesions around his mouth with surrounding erythema. He is well with no change in his oral intake. What is the most likely diagnosis?

a. Herpes simplex.
b. Dermatophytosis.
c. Impetigo.
d. Varicella zoster.

12) A 72-year-old female presents to her primary care doctor with a 1-day history of a burning sensation across the left side of her abdomen. On examination, you note clusters of vesicles in a dermatomal distribution that do not cross the midline of her abdomen. You diagnose shingles. How would you manage this condition?

a. Admit to hospital for intravenous antibiotics.
b. Oral acyclovir.
c. Analgesia only.
d. Oral antibiotics.

13) Which one of the following is considered pathognomonic for alopecia areata?

a. Skin scarring.
b. Broken hairs.
c. Exclamation mark hairs.
d. Scales on the scalp.

14) A 50-year-old female presents to her primary care doctor with facial flushing that she is finding socially embarrassing. On examination, she has erythema, telangiectasia and pinpoint pustules across her nose and cheeks. She has noticed the flushing is worse when she goes into a warm room and when she drinks alcohol. What is the most likely diagnosis?

a. Alcohol-related skin changes.
b. Acne vulgaris.
c. Seborrheic dermatitis.
d. Rosacea.

15) An 18-year-old female who has just moved away from home to university is brought to the emergency department by her housemates, drowsy with a fever and headache. On examination, she looks unwell and you note her skin is mottled with spreading purpuric lesions. What would be your initial management of this patient?

a. IV ceftriaxone.
b. IV acyclovir.
c. IV co-amoxiclav.
d. Lumbar puncture.

16) A 23-year-old male attends the outpatient dermatology clinic for review of his chronic plaque psoriasis. He is keen to know more about his condition and asks you which cell mediates his autoimmune disorder. What would you tell him?

a. B-cells.
b. Natural killer cells.
c. Macrophages.
d. T-cells.

17) A 19-year-old male develops brown, hard, tender lumps on the soles of his feet diagnosed as keratoderma blennorrhagicum. He reports an episode of joint swelling, red eyes and burning on passing urine 6 weeks ago. Which HLA gene is most commonly associated with this condition?

a. HLA DR3.
b. HLA B27.
c. HLA DQ2.
d. HLA B47.

18) A 23-year-old female presents to her primary care doctor with problematic excess hair. She is fair-haired but reports dark facial hair around her chin. On further questioning, her periods are infrequent, she is not taking any contraception and is not sexually active. She has no family history. On examination, she is obese and there is evidence of hirsutism. What is the most likely cause of her hirsutism?

a. Polycystic ovary syndrome.
b. Congenital adrenal hyperplasia.
c. Idiopathic hirsutism.
d. Androgen-secreting tumour.

19) A 72-year-old male presents to the dermatology clinic with a lesion on the side of his nose that has been present for several years. Clinically you suspect that the lesion may be a basal cell carcinoma. Which of the following is not typically found on examination of a basal cell carcinoma?

a. Pearly colour.
b. Tender on palpation.
c. Telangiectasia across the surface.
d. Rolled edge.

20) A 55-year-old female presents to her primary care doctor with an itchy, red rash around her left nipple. On examination, there are scaly plaques on the left nipple and surrounding skin and you note a bloody discharge. She has a past medical history of hypertension and eczema as a child but "grew out of it". What is the most likely cause of her rash?

a. Cellulitis.
b. Eczema.
c. Paget's disease of the breast.
d. Melanoma.

21) A 6-year-old boy is brought to the primary care doctor by his mother concerned that he has been unwell for the last couple of days. The mother reports low-grade fever, reduced appetite and noticed today a pink rash that started behind his ears and is now spreading down his body. The child is normally fit and well; his parents do not believe in vaccinating their children. On examination, you

note that the child looks fairly well and his temperature is 37.7°C. There is a pink macular rash which has spread to the child's trunk and palpable cervical lymphadenopathy. What is the most likely diagnosis?

a. Scarlet fever.
b. Chickenpox.
c. Rubella.
d. Measles.

22) A 48-year-old female is in the intensive care unit with septic shock requiring inotropic support; she receives the first intravenous dose of her antibiotics as a bolus. Within 10 minutes she develops severe flushing and erythema to the whole of her upper body; it is not urticarial and there is no evidence of anaphylaxis. You suspect red man syndrome. Which of the following antibiotics is most likely to have caused this?

a. Flucloxacillin.
b. Vancomycin.
c. Clarithromycin.
d. Metronidazole.

23) A 20-year-old female is referred to the dermatology outpatient clinic by her primary care doctor due to recurrent unexplained skin rashes. Her primary care doctor has thoroughly investigated her and found no notable abnormalities; the symptoms have not improved with a variety of treatments including emollients, topical steroids and topical antibiotics. She has recently commenced sertraline. On examination, you note a

superficial geometric pattern of lesions on her forearms. What is the most likely diagnosis?

a.   Contact dermatitis.
b.   Eczema.
c.   Seborrheic dermatitis.
d.   Dermatitis artefacta.

Extended matching questions

Itching

a. Eczema.
b. Primary biliary cirrhosis.
c. Uraemia.
d. Iron deficiency anaemia.

e. Hyperthyroidism.
f. Hypothyroidism.
g. Hodgkin's lymphoma.
h. Diabetes mellitus.

Match the clinical description to the most likely cause of itching.

1) A 45-year-old female with fatigue and severe itching, with blood tests showing anti-mitochondrial antibodies.

2) A 58-year-old male with itching who you notice on examination has an arteriovenous fistula.

3) A 48-year-old female complaining of a swelling in the neck, itching and heat intolerance.

4) A 78-year-old male complaining of shortness of breath, itching and altered bowel habit.

5) A 22-year-old female complaining of itching and a lump in her neck which when examined feels rubbery.

Systemic disease

a.	Coeliac disease.	e.	Aortic stenosis.
b.	Systemic lupus erythematosus.	f.	Diabetes mellitus.
c.	Hyperthyroidism.	g.	Scleroderma.
d.	Sarcoidosis.	h.	Chronic liver disease.

Match the clinical description of the skin rash to the systemic disease that most likely causes the dermatological manifestation.

6) Tender, red discrete nodules present bilaterally on the shins.

7) Multiple small lesions present on the trunk with blood vessels radiating outwards which blanch on pressure. Patients may also have reddening of the palms.

8) Hyperpigmented, hyperkeratotic skin described as feeling like velvet.

9) A rash across the bridge of the nose and across the cheeks, sparing the nasolabial folds.

10) Profoundly itchy papules and vesicles found in symmetrical distribution on the extensor surfaces of the elbow.

Nail changes

a.	Splinter haemorrhages.	e.	Terry's nails.
b.	Nail pitting.	f.	Finger clubbing.
c.	Beau's lines.	g.	Linear melanonychia.
d.	Koilonychia.	h.	Paronychia.

Match the clinical description to the nail change.

11) This nail change is often described as looking 'spoon-shaped' and may be seen in iron deficiency anaemia.

12) A typically white nail that is often seen in liver cirrhosis.

13) May be seen in infective endocarditis.

14) A descriptive term of subungual melanoma.

15) A nail change commonly seen in patients with psoriasis.

Childhood rashes

a. Measles.

b. Scarlet fever.

c. Scalded skin syndrome.

d. Impetigo.

e. Chickenpox.

f. Parvovirus B19.

g. Hand, foot and mouth disease.

h. Molluscum contagiosum.

Match the description of the disease that may present with a rash and found in children with the most likely diagnosis.

16) Characterised by multiple papules, typically pearly pink/red, with dimples in the centre.

17) The rash is typically red and feels like sandpaper; it may be associated with a strawberry tongue.

18) Another name for this disease is slapped cheek syndrome due to the red rash on the cheeks.

19) A superficial skin infection that classically has a honey-coloured crusting.

20) Features other than the rash include cough, coryza, conjunctivitis and Koplik spots.

Ulcers

a.	Venous ulcer.	e.	Vasculitic ulcer.
b.	Pressure ulcer.	f.	Pyoderma gangrenosum.
c.	Neuropathic ulcer.	g.	Bacterial infection-related ulcer.
d.	Diabetic ulcer.	h.	Arterial ulcer.

Match the clinical presentation with the most likely ulcer.

21) A 50-year-old obese male presents with an ulcer on the ball of his foot. Examination of his foot reveals a peripheral neuropathy. His HbA1c is 67.

22) A 67-year-old male with a well-demarcated ulcer on his lateral malleolus which is particularly painful at night. You cannot palpate his dorsalis pedis or posterior tibial pulse.

23) An 88-year-old nursing home resident with severe Alzheimer's disease presents with an ulcer on her sacrum. On examination, there is full-thickness tissue loss and you are able to see subcutaneous fat with a covering layer of slough.

24) A 56-year-old obese female, with varicosities on both legs has an ulcer present on her left inner ankle. She has a background of hypertension.

25) A 28-year-old female with loose stools and mouth ulcers presents with what was initially a small red lump on her leg which has rapidly progressed into a large, painful, purple-edged ulcer with an irregular border.

Neonatal dermatological diagnoses

a. Milia.

b. Strawberry naevus.

c. Erythema toxicum.

d. Mongolian blue spot.

e. Port-wine stain.

f. Non-accidental injury.

g. Seborrheic dermatitis.

h. Caput succedaneum.

Match the description of the skin change/rash found in the newborn or first few weeks of life.

26) A baby on his newborn examination is found to have a large blue macule over his buttocks.

27) If this is found on the face it may be a sign of Sturge-Weber syndrome.

28) Also known as milk spots.

29) A red, blotchy rash with pustules; it is benign and self-resolving.

30) Cradle cap is an example of this.

Fungal disease

a.   Tinea pedis.
b.   Pityriasis versicolor.
c.   Pityriasis rosea.
d.   Tinea capitis.

e.   Tinea unguium.
f.   Intertrigo.
g.   Tinea corporis.
h.   Candidiasis.

Match the description of a fungal infection to the most suitable diagnosis or organism.

31) Also known as athlete's foot.

32) Caused by *Malassezia*.

33) An invasive disease that can cause dysphagia in immunosuppressed patients.

34) Raised, scaly, red rings with central sparing found on the body.

35) Occurs in skin folds.

Eponymous signs

a. Auspitz's sign.

b. Pastia's sign.

c. Russell's sign.

d. Cullen's sign.

e. Grey-Turner's sign.

f. Gottron's sign.

g. Nikolsky's sign.

h. Hutchinson's sign.

Match the description of the examination finding to its eponymous name.

36) Scaly, red papules found in dermatomyositis.

37) Typically found in psoriasis, it is the appearance of pinpoint bleeding spots when scales are gently removed.

38) Superficial bruising around the umbilicus that may be caused by acute pancreatitis.

39) Refers to a callus on the back of the hand relating to self-induced vomiting.

40) A pigment band the length of the nail bed involving the adjacent nail fold.

Dermatology in pregnancy

a.	Striae gravidarum.	e.	Linea nigra.
b.	Telogen effluvium.	f.	Pemphigoid gestationis.
c.	Polymorphic eruption.	g.	Cholestatic pruritus.
d.	Melasma.	h.	Palmar erythema.

Match the clinical description to the dermatological condition found in pregnancy or puerperium.

41) Due to increased circulating levels of oestrogen. It is also found in liver cirrhosis.

42) A 24-year-old female gave birth to her first child 1 month previously. She is concerned as she has noticed that her hair is thinning which is particularly noticeable when she brushes her hair.

43) A 28-year-old female is 34 weeks pregnant. She reports intense itching. On examination, she is well and there are no signs other than scratch marks. Her bloods are unremarkable other than a mildly raised ALP.

44) A 36-year-old female develops dark macules on her face during pregnancy. She developed these during her last pregnancy and they resolved after she gave birth.

45) A dark, vertical band of hyperpigmented skin down the midline of the abdomen.

Short answer questions

1) A 24-year-old female presents to her primary care doctor with an itchy rash on her elbows and knees. She is fit and well normally. On questioning, she has had a recent relationship breakdown and is struggling with deadlines at work; she has started smoking again. On examination, there are well-demarcated pink plaques with a fine silver scale distributed symmetrically on extensor surfaces. You suspect plaque psoriasis; she states her sister has this.

a. State two risk factors for chronic plaque psoriasis that the patient has   2 marks
in the above history.

b. Give two signs that you may see on this patient's nails.   2 marks

c. Give three topical treatments that may be useful in the management   3 marks
of this patient's disease.

d. Chronic plaque psoriasis is a subtype of psoriasis; give two other   2 marks
subtypes of psoriasis.

e. What sign is described when pinpoint bleeding occurs when scales   1 mark
are gently scraped?

2) A 30-year-old female presents to her primary care doctor as she has seen a recent campaign advising people to get their moles checked. On examination, you find no concerning features. She is keen to learn more about skin cancer.

a. You inform the patient about the 'ABCDE' of signs for pigmented   5 marks
lesions; what do each of the letters stand for in this approach?

b. Give two risk factors for malignant melanoma.   2 marks

c. Give one subtype of malignant melanoma.   1 mark

d. Which staging system is used to classify malignant melanoma?   1 mark
e. What measurement is obtained upon biopsy which can be used to   1 mark
    predict outcomes of melanoma?

3) A 72-year-old male is admitted to the medical assessment
    unit with a red, hot and painful leg following an insect
    bite. He has a past medical history of angina, COPD and
    Type 2 diabetes; he is a current smoker. His regular
    medications include a GTN spray, metformin, gliclazide
    and insulin. Initially he is treated for cellulitis with oral
    antibiotics and analgesia. His pain intensifies and is not
    eased by analgesia. When you re-examine him he looks
    unwell; you notice the skin is discoloured and blistered.

a. Give four cardinal signs of inflammation.   4 marks
b. Give two organisms that commonly cause cellulitis.   2 marks
c. What is the most likely diagnosis in this patient?   1 mark
d. What in his history has predisposed this condition?   1 mark
e. Give four blood tests that should be taken in this patient.   2 marks

4) A 24-year-old male attends the emergency department
    after developing an itchy rash following accidental ingestion
    of a peanut; you are asked to urgently review him. On
    examination, there are red, raised wheals covering most of
    his body, his face appears swollen and his lips and tongue
    are protruding. It is difficult to observe his airway, you
    auscultate wheeze on his chest and he is hypotensive and
    tachycardic on review of his observations.

a. What is the rash described above and by what mechanism does it 2 marks
    occur?
b. Give three immediate medications that should be administered.   3 marks
c. Which team would it be appropriate to refer this patient to upon 2 marks
    discharge and give one investigation they may perform?

d. Give two pieces of advice you would give on discharge.   2 marks

e. Give one non-allergic drug reaction that can cause angioedema.   1 mark

5) An 18-year-old female attends her primary care doctor complaining of an intensely itchy rash which has developed on the extensor surfaces of her elbows. On examination, there are papules and vesicles present bilaterally on clusters on the patient's elbows with scratch marks. On further questioning, she reports intermittent loose stools, abdominal pain and distension for the last 2 months for which she has been meaning to seek medical advice.

a. What is the most likely cause of this patient's diarrhoea?   1 mark

b. What is characteristically seen on biopsy of the skin lesions?   1 mark

c. Give two different managements of dermatitis herpetiformis.   2 marks

d. Give eight blood tests that should be performed in this patient. 4 marks

e. Name two autoimmune diseases that are associated with dermatitis 2 marks
    herpetiformis.

6) A 52-year-old male presents to the primary care doctor alongside his wife who made an appointment for him as she is concerned about his alcohol intake. He drinks one 750ml bottle of 13.5% wine per night. He has been under stress at work recently, he denies any significant past medical history and your physical examination is unremarkable.

a. Calculate how many units of alcohol he is drinking per week.   1 mark

b. You use the CAGE questionnaire to assess for problem drinking; what 2 marks
    are the four questions that make up this test?

c. Give four skin findings that you may see on examination of a patient 4 marks
    with liver disease.

d. Give two nail changes that you may see on examination of a patient   2 marks
   with liver disease.

e. Which breakdown compound of ethanol causes flushing.   1 mark

7) A 16-year-old female attends her primary care doctor concerned about her skin; she is teary and states she wears a lot of make-up to try to cover up her skin. She has no significant past medical history and takes no regular medications. After examining her you diagnose moderate acne vulgaris.

a. Give three skin lesions that may be found on examination in acne.   3 marks

b. She is keen to commence medication; give three different   3 marks
   medications that can be used in primary care in the management of
   acne.

c. Unfortunately, her acne does not improve on initial management and   1 mark
   she attends a dermatologist who commences isotretinoin. What
   category of medication does this belong to?

d. Give two complications of acne vulgaris.   2 marks

e. If the patient was a hirsute, overweight female with irregular,   1 mark
   infrequent periods, what underlying diagnosis would you consider?

8) A 34-year-old male presents to his primary care doctor with a rash on his leg. On examination, there is a red rash with central sparing which has a target appearance, he denies any other symptoms and feels well in himself. He is a keen traveller and reports a recent tick bite on holiday in America at the site of the rash. You suspect the patient may have Lyme disease.

a. What is the name of the rash described above?   1 mark

b. Which bacteria causes the above and what type is this?   3 marks

c. Give two features of early disseminated Lyme disease.   2 marks

d. You commence doxycycline; 2 hours later he develops a headache, 2 marks
    myalgia and chills. He is not allergic to doxycycline. What is the most
    likely cause of his symptoms?

e. Give two pieces of advice you would give the patient to try to prevent 2 marks
    further tick bites.

9) A 5-year-old child is an inpatient on the paediatric ward
    with suspected Kawasaki disease; he initially presented
    unwell and pyrexial with dermatological changes. His
    mother states he is normally fit and well, is up to date
    with his vaccinations and has no medical problems or
    medications.

a. Give three skin/mucous membrane changes for Kawasaki disease. 3 marks
b. Give three differential diagnoses of Kawasaki disease. 3 marks
c. On day 5 he is given an IV therapy; what is this likely to be? 1 mark
d. Which oral medication do you commence him on? 1 mark
e. Why is it important that he is monitored with echocardiograms? 2 marks

10) A medical student is on attachment in dermatology during
    clinic; preliminary questions are put to the student to
    prepare them for clinic.

a. The skin has many functions; name four of these. 4 marks
b. What three layers is the skin made up of? 3 marks
c. What is the function of fibroblasts? 1 mark
d. Give one subtype of sweat gland. 1 mark
e. Which sensory receptor is responsible for sensing deep pressure and 1 mark
    vibration?

11) A 26-year-old female attends her primary care doctor concerned about patches of hair loss at the front and side of her scalp. She has worn hair extensions for cosmetic reasons since her teenage years. You find the 'fringe' sign on examination of her scalp. She is normally fit and well and denies any significant past medical history; she takes no regular medications.

a. What are the three stages of hair follicle growth? 3 marks
b. What is the most likely cause of this patient's hair loss? 1 mark
c. Give two complications that may occur in this patient. 2 marks
d. Give three examples of dermatological disease that can cause 3 marks reversible hair thinning or patchy hair loss.
e. A 32-year-old male attends clinic concerned his hair is thinning; you 1 mark diagnose androgenetic alopecia male pattern. Name one drug therapy you could start in this patient.

12) A 19-year-old male attends his primary care doctor with an itchy rash in the flexural surfaces of his elbows; he is struggling to sleep due to the itch and feels his skin is dry. On further questioning, he has a past medical history of eczema that he thought he had "grown out of as a child" and has recently changed washing power since moving out of his parent's house. He has a positive family history of atopy. You suspect he is experiencing an eczema flare.

a. What is atopy? 1 mark
b. Give two other atopic medical conditions this patient may have. 2 marks
c. Give four common trigger factors for eczema. 4 marks
d. Give two initial management plans for this patient's eczema. 2 marks
e. He presents to the emergency department several months later after 1 mark marked worsening of his eczema and escalation of treatment with a generalised redness of the skin; he is hypothermic and looks unwell. Which complication of eczema is most likely to have occurred?

13) A 72-year-old male presents to his primary care doctor with a lesion on his ear that his daughter is concerned about; he cannot remember how long it has been there but it has been present "for a while". On examination, there is a thickened plaque with a scaly surface on his right ear; he doesn't think it has changed in the last couple of months. He reports a past medical history of basal cell carcinoma which was removed 5 years ago, previous prolonged sun exposure from when he used to live in Spain and hypertension. You suspect a premalignant condition.

a. What is the most likely cause of this premalignant condition? 1 mark

b. If there was clinical uncertainty regarding the diagnosis, what 1 mark investigation would you order?

c. You provide the patient with reassurance that it is unlikely to be 3 marks malignant; however, he is keen to have the lesion removed. Give three different ways that this could be treated.

d. This patient had a previous basal cell carcinoma. Give three features 3 marks you would find on examination of a typical nodular basal cell carcinoma.

e. Give two pieces of advice you would give to a patient to reduce their 2 marks risk of developing skin cancer.

Chapter 2

Obstetrics & gynaecology
QUESTIONS

Single best answer questions

1) What percentage of those trying to conceive will be successful in 1 year?

a.   75%.
b.   84%.
c.   95%.
d.   65%.

2) Which of the following is not considered a risk factor for pelvic inflammatory disease?

a.   Multiple sexual partners.
b.   Previous diagnosis of endometriosis.
c.   Presence of an intrauterine device.
d.   Previous treatment for an STI.

3)   Which of the following is not a complication of gestational diabetes?

a.   Shoulder dystocia.
b.   Miscarriage.
c.   Polyhydramnios.
d.   Intrauterine growth restriction.

4)   Which of the following can be used in overactive bladder syndrome?

a.   Anticholinergics.
b.   Alpha-blockers.
c.   Antimuscarinics.
d.   H2 antagonists.

5)   Which of the following is not a recognised complication of pre-eclampsia?

a.   Seizure.
b.   Cerebral haemorrhage.
c.   Intrauterine growth restriction.
d.   Macrosomia.

6)   Which hormone peaks just prior to ovulation?

a.   LH.
b.   FSH.
c.   Oestrogen.
d.   Progesterone.

7) Which of the following is a risk factor for Down's syndrome?

a. Low maternal age.
b. Low PAPP-A.
c. Obesity.
d. Cocaine use.

8) At which gestation is rubella most likely to cause fetal abnormality?

a. 8-10 weeks.
b. 11-16 weeks.
c. 16-24 weeks.
d. >24 weeks.

9) What is the pathogenesis of lichen sclerosis?

a. Viral.
b. Autoimmune.
c. Bacterial.
d. Neoplastic.

10) Which of the following is a method of emergency contraception?

a. Mirena IUS.
b. Combined contraceptive pill.
c. Copper IUD.
d. Depo-Provera injection.

11) Which of the following is less frequently elevated in obstetric cholestasis?

a.   Bile acids.
b.   Bilirubin.
c.   AST.
d.   ALT.

12) Which of the following is not associated with maternal hypothyroidism?

a.   Neurodevelopmental delay.
b.   Microcephaly.
c.   Miscarriage.
d.   Subfertility.

13) Which of the following is not a risk factor for cervical cancer?

a.   Increased number of sexual partners.
b.   Immunosuppression.
c.   Smoking.
d.   Early menarche.

14) Which type of ovarian tumour is associated with CA19-9?

a.   Mucinous.
b.   Dysgerminoma.
c.   Endometrioid.
d.   Sertoli-Leydig.

15) Which of the following antihypertensives is unsafe in breastfeeding?

a. Labetalol.
b. Captopril.
c. Ramipril.
d. Nifedipine.

16) Which of the following is not a fetal complication of toxoplasmosis in pregnancy?

a. Blindness.
b. Macrosomia.
c. Hepatosplenomegaly.
d. Intercranial calcification.

17) Which gene is most associated with ovarian cancer?

a. BRCA-1.
b. BRCA-2.
c. Lynch G1.
d. CFTR.

18) Which type of twins is associated with twin-twin transfusion?

a. Monochorionic monoamniotic.
b. Monochorionic diamniotic.
c. Diamniotic monoamniotic.
d. Diamniotic diamniotic.

19) Which of the following hormones increases in menopause?

a. FSH.
b. Oestrogen.
c. Progesterone.
d. Testosterone.

20) Which antibiotic is recommended intrapartum for women with known Group B *Streptococcus*?

a. Benzylpenicillin.
b. Flucloxacillin.
c. Amoxicillin.
d. Co-amoxiclav.

21) Which of the following analgesics should not be used in pregnancy?

a. Paracetamol.
b. Codeine phosphate.
c. Morphine sulphate.
d. Ibuprofen.

22) Which of the following is not a common site for endometriosis?

a. Pouch of Douglas.
b. Uterosacral ligaments.
c. Anterior aspect of the bladder.
d. Ovaries.

23) Which of the following is a complete contraindication to the combined contraceptive pill?

a.   History of DVT.
b.   Migraine.
c.   Hypertension.
d.   Raised BMI.

Extended matching questions

Antepartum haemorrhage

a. Placenta praevia.
b. Cervical carcinoma.
c. Vaginal candidiasis.
d. Placental abruption.

e. Vasa praevia.
f. Cervical polyp.
g. Cervical ectropion.
h. Ectopic pregnancy.

Match the description of the patient with the most likely diagnosis.

1) A 34-week pregnant female presents with abdominal pain and vaginal bleeding following a road traffic accident.

2) A 26-week pregnant female presents with small amounts of vaginal bleeding; she had had some postcoital bleeding prior to pregnancy and her last smear test showed the presence of endometrial cells.

3) A 39-week pregnant female presents with intermittent abdominal pain and uterine contractions. When her membranes rupture, a large quantity of frank blood is seen.

4) A female presents at around 9 weeks pregnant with vaginal bleeding and left-sided abdominal pain.

5) A 38-week pregnant female presents with massive vaginal bleeding and intermittent abdominal pain associated with uterine tightening. She has missed several scheduled ultrasound appointments and has had several episodes of vaginal bleeding during the pregnancy.

Postnatal vaginal discharge

a. Retained placenta.   e. Candida.
b. Endometritis.   f. Normal lochia.
c. Chlamydia infection.   g. Menstruation.
d. Rectovaginal fistula.   h. Cervical cancer.

Match the description of the patient with the most likely diagnosis.

6) A female who is 4 days postpartum presents with increased vaginal bleeding and a fever. On examination, she is tachycardic and her temperature is 38.4°C.

7) A female who is 8 weeks postnatal, artificially feeding her baby, presents with vaginal bleeding. There is no foul odour and her observations are stable.

8) A female who is 1 week postnatal presents with a foul-smelling discharge vaginally; during her delivery she suffered a third-degree tear. On questioning, she states she has been passing some gas per vagina.

9) A female who is 9 days postnatal presents because she is still passing some red/brown discharge following the birth of her baby.

10) A female who is 6 months postnatal has presented with a white vaginal discharge and some vulval irritation.

Benign pelvic masses

a.	Luteal cyst.	e.	Ovarian fibroma.
b.	Fibroid uterus.	f.	Polycystic ovary syndrome.
c.	Ovarian torsion.	g.	Endometrioma.
d.	Dermoid cyst.	h.	Pregnancy.

Match the description of the patient with the most likely diagnosis.

11) A 25-year-old female presents with an incidental finding on an ultrasound scan, whilst being investigated for menorrhagia, of a 20 x 15 x 17mm fluid-filled cyst on the right ovary.

12) A 45-year-old female presents with a history of a gradual onset of abdominal bloating and increasing breathlessness (worse on lying flat). An ultrasound scan shows a solid mass around the left ovary.

13) A 32-year-old female presents to the primary care doctor with a palpable mass on her left side. She is referred to the gynaecologist and when the mass is excised it is found to contain hair and teeth.

14) A 27-year-old female presents to her primary care doctor with ongoing pelvic pain, which is worse around the time of menstruation. An ultrasound scan reveals a unilocular cyst on her left ovary, which shows a ground-glass appearance.

15) A 44-year-old female presents with abdominal bloating, menorrhagia and urinary frequency.

Secondary amenorrhoea

a.   Prolactinoma.
b.   Polycystic ovary syndrome.
c.   Hypothalamic dysfunction.
d.   Sheehan's syndrome.

e.   Hyperthyroidism.
f.   Premature ovarian failure.
g.   Cervical stenosis.
h.   Hypothyroidism.

Match the description of the patient with the most likely diagnosis.

16) A 21-year-old student presents with amenorrhoea for the last 6 months. She has recently been diagnosed with depression following failure of her exams.

17) A 32-year-old female presents with amenorrhoea, 12 months following the birth of her child. She has not recommenced her menses since the birth. She had a 2L postpartum haemorrhage while delivering and required three units of blood.

18) A 26-year-old female presents with amenorrhoea and lower abdominal pain 6 months following a LLETZ procedure for abnormal cervical cells.

19) A 36-year-old female presents with amenorrhoea for the last 8 months. She has also been complaining of headaches and was involved in a road traffic accident 2 weeks ago.

20) A 29-year-old female attends her primary care doctor complaining of palpitations, tremor and amenorrhoea.

Vulval lesions

a.	Vulval interstitial neoplasia.	e.	Lichen sclerosis.
b.	Lichen planus.	f.	Psoriasis.
c.	Paget's disease of the vulva.	g.	Herpes simplex.
d.	Squamous cell carcinoma.	h.	HPV.

Match the description of the patient with the most likely diagnosis.

21) A 24-year-old female presents with a painful ulcer on her labia minora. She has recently returned from Thailand where she has been travelling for 6 months.

22) A 65-year-old female presents to her primary care doctor complaining of vulval pruritus. On examination, there are bilateral white shiny patches on the labia majora and the labia minora have shrunk significantly.

23) A 55-year-old female presents with a well-defined, scaly lesion on her vulva. She has just undergone a mastectomy for breast cancer.

24) A 28-year-old female presents for colposcopy following an abnormal smear test. She had a biopsy which showed CIN 2. The nurse who performed the examination noticed a 15mm lesion on her labia minora.

25) A 36-year-old female presents to her primary care doctor complaining of a smooth lesion on her labia majora. She also has some scaly lesions on the extensor surface of her elbows.

Chromosomal abnormalities

a.	Turner syndrome.	e.	Klinefelter syndrome.
b.	Down's syndrome.	f.	Sheehan syndrome.
c.	Androgen insensitivity.	g.	Kallmann syndrome.
d.	McCune-Albright syndrome.	h.	Müllerian agenesis.

Match the presentation to the condition.

26) Phenotypically female, blind-ended vagina, absent cervix and uterus, normal breasts, testes seen intra-abdominally.

27) Azoospermia, phenotypically male and no secondary sexual characteristics.

28) Phenotypically female, poor secondary sexual characteristics, infertility and anosmia.

29) Phenotypically female, short stature, webbed neck and hypoplastic nails and 4th metacarpals.

30) Phenotypically and genotypically female, absent vagina and uterus, normal external genitalia, ovaries present and renal abnormalities.

Ovarian malignancies

a.	Mucinous.	e.	Teratoma.
b.	Choriocarcinoma.	f.	Serous.
c.	Endometrioma.	g.	Granulosa cell.
d.	Dysgerminoma.	h.	Thecoma.

Match the features to the type of tumour.

31) Most common type of epithelial ovarian tumour.

32) Could be associated with pseudomyxoma.

33) Benign and associated with Meigs syndrome.

34) Solid unilateral ovarian tumour with raised β-HCG.

35) Associated with chromosomal abnormalities.

Spermatogenesis

a.	Sertoli cells.	e.	Spermatid.
b.	LH.	f.	Leydig cells.
c.	FSH.	g.	Spermatocyte.
d.	Testosterone.	h.	Spermatogonia.

Match the most appropriate answer with the stages of spermatogenesis.

36) In which cell does the mitotic division of the male gamete occur?

37) In which cell does androgen production occur?

38) Mitosis occurs under the influence of which hormone?

39) Which hormone transforms spermatids into sperm?

40) What is the name of the primary cell type in spermatogenesis?

Congenital malformations

a.	Tetralogy of Fallot.	e.	Ventricular septal defect.
b.	Coarctation of the aorta.	f.	Gastroschisis.
c.	Spina bifida cystica.	g.	Spina bifida occulta.
d.	Exomphalos.	h.	Patent ductus arteriosus.

Match the description with the most likely abnormality.

41) A baby is born with its bowel protruding from its abdominal wall which is not covered in peritoneum.

42) A baby is born and during its neonatal check is found to have a higher blood pressure in the arms than legs.

43) A midwife notices a small hairy patch on the back, whilst weighing an otherwise healthy baby.

44) A baby is 2 days postnatal and during the routine baby check a continuous machine-like murmur is found and the feet are noted to be slightly cyanosed.

45) A baby is noted shortly after birth to be turning blue and becoming limp when crying; the fingers are also noted to be clubbed.

Short answer questions

1) A 26-year-old female attends her primary care doctor seeking advice on conception. She has a past medical history of epilepsy. She has not been pregnant previously and would like some advice regarding her medication.

a. Name four fetal and neonatal complications associated with antiepileptic drugs in pregnancy. 4 marks

b. Give two complications of stopping antiepileptic drugs. 2 marks

c. What drug should be prescribed to prevent fetal complications? Include a name and dosage. 2 marks

d. What will happen to antiepileptic drug levels during pregnancy? 1 mark

e. What is the advice regarding breastfeeding? 1 mark

2) A 45-year-old female attends a clinic complaining of heavy periods for the last 6 months. Previously she has been regular with a cycle length of 28 days. She is currently sexually active using contraceptive barrier methods.

a. What is the definition of menorrhagia? 1 mark

b. Name two causes of menorrhagia, one systemic and one local. 2 marks

c. Name one feature in a history suggestive of significant menorrhagia. 1 mark

d. What investigations can be performed to assess the cause of significant menorrhagia (one serum and one physical)? 2 marks

e. Name four medical methods of managing menorrhagia (two requiring contraception, two without). 4 marks

3) A 25-year-old female attends her primary care doctor complaining of severe premenstrual abdominal/pelvic pain. She also experiences pain during intercourse. Her menses are regular and of normal flow.

a. What is the definition of endometriosis?   1 mark
b. Explain the implantation theory as a cause of endometriosis.   2 marks
c. Name two common sites for endometriosis.   2 marks
d. What is the method of diagnosis for endometriosis?   1 mark
e. Name four treatments for endometriosis.   4 marks

4) A 70-year-old female has been referred to the 2-week wait clinic with a 3-month history of weight loss of 10kg and general abdominal bloating.

a. Name three serum tumour markers that should be performed.   3 marks
b. Name one gene associated with ovarian malignancy.   1 mark
c. Name two risk factors for ovarian malignancy.   2 marks
d. What are the three broad types of malignant ovarian tumours?   3 marks
e. Name one common site for metastasis.   1 mark

5) A 60-year-old female attends her primary care doctor complaining of a mass that appears to be arising from her vagina. She is also experiencing some urinary incontinence when straining, coughing and sneezing.

a. What is the term used for this type of incontinence?   1 mark
b. Name the three muscles in the pelvic floor.   3 marks
c. Specify two risk factors that are associated with uterovaginal prolapse.   2 marks
d. What can be done to prevent prolapse?   2 marks
e. State one conservative and one surgical treatment that can be offered.   2 marks

6) A 26-year-old female attends her routine antenatal check-up at 28 weeks. The fundal height is found to be low for her dates and an ultrasound scan is performed. The results indicate an abnormally small amount of amniotic fluid surrounding the fetus.

a. State one acute and one chronic cause of oligohydramnios.   2 marks
b. Specify two fetal complications that can occur post-delivery.   2 marks
c. Name two potential complications that could occur during delivery. 2 marks
d. State the measurement for oligohydramnios and how it is taken.   2 marks
e. Name two methods to treat oligohydramnios.   2 marks

7) You have been called to review a patient in the maternity day assessment unit who is complaining of headache. She is 32 weeks pregnant and this is her first pregnancy. She is noted to have a blood pressure of 160/110mmHg.

a. State three other symptoms that you would specifically ask about.   3 marks
b. Name two investigations you should perform at this stage.   2 marks
c. What is the definition of pre-eclampsia?   1 mark
d. What other syndrome is associated with pre-eclampsia?   1 mark
e. State three features of this syndrome.   3 marks

8) A female presents with painful uterine contractions which are occurring every 3 minutes. She is at 40 weeks' gestation and this is her first pregnancy. She is examined and is found to have a fully effaced cervix with 3cm dilatation.

a.   Define the three stages of labour.   3 marks
b.   How fast would you expect cervical dilatation to occur from this point 1 mark
     onwards?
c.   Give three analgesia types used in labour.   3 marks
d.   What is the anatomical landmark that is used to determine the 1 mark
     station of the fetal head when examining internally?
e.   Describe two methods of management of the third stage of labour.   2 marks

9)   A 43-year-old female attends the consultant-led antenatal
     clinic at 13 weeks pregnant. She had her dating scan the
     week before. This was an unplanned pregnancy and she
     already has three children, the youngest being 10 years
     old. She has been found to be high risk for chromosomal
     abnormalities from the combined screening test.

a.   What are the components of the combined screening test?   4 marks
b.   Which three conditions does the combined screening test for and 3 marks
     what are the chromosomal abnormalities for each?
c.   Name a method of invasive testing for a definitive diagnosis.   1 mark
d.   This test comes back as abnormal and she wishes to terminate the 1 mark
     pregnancy. What method would be used at this gestation?
e.   What blood test is important to do when doing this and why?   1 mark

10) A 30-year-old female and her partner attend a fertility
     clinic. They have been trying to conceive for 18 months
     and have so far been unsuccessful.

a.   What is the definition of infertility?   1 mark
b.   In the male, name two medical conditions that may reduce fertility. 2 marks
c.   Name a cause for subfertility in this patient in the following three 3 marks
     categories — ovulatory dysfunction, tubal factor and uterine problem.
d.   Specify two types of imaging used to investigate female infertility. 2 marks
e.   Give two features measured in semen analysis.   2 marks

11) A 25-year-old female presents with severe vomiting at around 12 weeks' gestation. She has not yet had her dating scan. A scan is requested, which shows a uterus that is larger than expected for dates and contains some grape-like vesicles and no evidence of a foetus.

a. What first-line antiemetic is used in hyperemesis gravidarum? 1 mark
b. Name and describe the development of the two types of hydatidiform 4 marks
moles.
c. Which serum test is elevated in molar pregnancy? 1 mark
d. Name the two types of neoplastic disease that can occur from a molar 2 marks
pregnancy.
e. What is the initial treatment and follow-up for molar pregnancy? 2 marks

12) A female is in the second stage of labour, following induction of labour at 37 weeks' gestation for growth above the 95th centile. The midwife pulls the emergency buzzer, you arrive in the room and she tells you that the head has delivered but there is a delay in the delivery of the body.

a. State the definition of shoulder dystocia. 3 marks
b. Specify one maternal, one fetal and one interventional risk factor 3 marks
which can predispose to shoulder dystocia.
c. Name the first two manoeuvres that should be employed to manage 2 marks
shoulder dystocia.
d. State one fetal complication of shoulder dystocia. 1 mark
e. Give one maternal complication of shoulder dystocia. 1 mark

13) A female who is currently 7 weeks pregnant attends her primary care doctor's practice with her 4-year-old son who has just contracted chicken pox whilst at nursery. The woman has not had chicken pox previously and was not vaccinated in her previous pregnancy.

a.   What is the incubation period of varicella zoster?   1 mark

b.   State three features of congenital varicella syndrome.   3 marks

c.   How is varicella zoster spread?   2 marks

d.   What type of vaccine is the varicella zoster vaccine and would it be   2 marks
     useful to give this patient this vaccine?

e.   What treatment would you give this woman and what route should it   2 marks
     be given by?

Chapter 3

Oncology
QUESTIONS

Single best answer questions

1) Which of the following antiemetics acts on the chemoreceptor trigger zone and increases gastric motility?

a. Haloperidol.
b. Cyclizine.
c. Metoclopramide.
d. Ondansetron.

2) Exposure to which of the following is most associated with the development of mesothelioma?

a. Blue asbestos.
b. White asbestos.
c. Brown asbestos.
d. Smoking.

3) A patient presents with blood mixed in the stool and significant weight loss. A colonoscopy shows a suspicious lesion in the sigmoid colon. The tumour has breached the mucosal and serosal layers; when resected the lymph nodes are not affected. How would you classify this tumour?

a.   Dukes A.
b.   Dukes B.
c.   Dukes C.
d.   Dukes D.

4) A patient is seen in their primary care practice with symptoms and signs consistent with Horner's syndrome. They are later proven to have an apical lung cancer (Pancoast's tumour). Which of the below are not associated with Horner's syndrome?

a.   Miosis.
b.   Anhidrosis.
c.   Ptosis.
d.   Mydriasis.

5) Which of the following breast tumours is not malignant in nature?

a.   Ductal carcinoma.
b.   Ductal papilloma.
c.   Mucinous carcinoma.
d.   Ductal carcinoma *in situ*.

6) Which of the following are not used to risk stratify men presenting with prostate cancer not extending into the capsule?

a. PSA.
b. Symptoms experienced.
c. Gleason score.
d. Tumour staging.

7) Which of these is a benign tumour of small muscle cells?

a. Chondroma.
b. Lipoma.
c. Rhabdomyoma.
d. Leiomyoma.

8) From which origin cell does an oligodendroglioma originate?

a. Glial cell.
b. Arachnoid cell.
c. Primitive neuroectodermal cell.
d. Nerve sheath cell.

9) When considering basal cell carcinoma which statement is false?

a. Very common.
b. Very invasive locally.
c. Metastasise frequently.
d. Usually occurs on the face.

10) When considering malignant melanoma what feature best reflects the chance of cure at the time of excision?

a. Length of time it has been present.
b. Patient age.
c. Lesion size.
d. Lesion depth (Breslow thickness).

11) Hydatidiform moles are a disorder of pregnancy; which of the following is not associated with the development of a molar pregnancy?

a. Large for dates uterus.
b. Bleeding in early pregnancy.
c. Abdominal pain.
d. Miscarriage.

12) Which of the following types of ovarian cancer is associated with pseudomyxoma peritonei?

a. Mucinous tumour.
b. Teratoma.
c. Dysgerminoma.
d. Granulosa cell tumour.

13) What is the most common presenting symptom for renal cell carcinoma?

a. Haematuria.
b. Loin pain.
c. Weight loss.
d. Dysuria.

14) What should be offered first to patients with metastatic prostate cancer?

a. LH analogue.
b. Chemotherapy.
c. Radiotherapy.
d. Bisphosphonate.

15) Which is associated with ~70% cases of hepatocellular carcinoma?

a. Alcoholic cirrhosis.
b. Hepatitis B or C infection.
c. Primary biliary cirrhosis.
d. Haemochromatosis.

16) Which of these is not a common risk factor for head and neck cancer?

a. Smoking.
b. Chewing betel nuts.
c. HPV exposure.
d. Obesity.

17) A 56-year-old male is treated with chemotherapy for a germ cell tumour. He develops tumour lysis syndrome. Which of the following biochemical abnormalities does not occur with tumour lysis syndrome?

a. Hypocalcaemia.
b. Hyperphosphataemia.
c. Hyperkalaemia.
d. Hypomagnesaemia.

18) The replacement of one mature cell type with another mature cell type is the definition of which of the following?

a. Dysplasia.
b. Metaplasia.
c. Neoplasia.
d. Hyperplasia.

19) A 62-year-old male with known prostate cancer presents with confusion. He is known to have bony metastasis in the spine. He has 5/5 power in his upper and lower limbs. What is the most important treatment?

a. Dexamethasone.
b. Intravenous fluids.
c. Radiotherapy.
d. Bisphosphonate.

20) Which of the following processes is not a typical hallmark of cancerous cells?

a. Introducing angiogenesis.
b. Evading immune destruction.
c. Resisting cell death.
d. Inability of cells to undergo apoptosis.

21) Which of the following syndromes is directly associated with the development of oesophageal adenocarcinoma?

a. Plummer-Vinson syndrome.
b. Zollinger-Ellison syndrome.
c. Down's syndrome.
d. Lynch syndrome.

22) A 54-year-old female presents to the emergency department with a change in behaviour, memory loss and right-sided hemiplegia. She is found to have a glioma. Where is its likely location?

a. Left frontal lobe.
b. Right frontal lobe.
c. Right occipital lobe.
d. Left temporal lobe.

23) A patient is receiving radical radiotherapy to the prostate bed following a prostatectomy. Which of the following is a likely side effect of the radiotherapy?

a. Dysuria.
b. Haematuria.
c. Diarrhoea.
d. Penile discharge.

Extended matching questions

Tumour markers

a. AFP.   e. Calcitonin.
b. CA125.   f. CEA.
c. CA19-9.   g. CA15-3.
d. PSA.   h. β-HCG.

Which tumour marker can be used to monitor the following cancers?

1) Used to monitor and aid the diagnosis of ovarian cancer.

2) Used to monitor colorectal cancer.

3) Used to monitor choriocarcinoma.

4) Used to monitor non-seminomatous germ cell cancers.

5) Used to monitor medullary cell carcinoma of the thyroid.

Technical terms used in oncology

a. Residual disease.

b. Disease-free survival.

c. Overall survival.

d. Progressive disease.

e. Complete response.

f. Partial response.

g. Remission rate.

h. Stable disease.

Which of the above terms best describes each definition?

6) Disappearance of all of the target lesions.

7) A 20% increase in the sum of the largest diameter target lesions.

8) The length of time after treatment for cancer with no signs and symptoms of disease.

9) Disease left at completion of planned treatment.

10) The percentage of patients alive at 5 years after diagnosis and treatment.

Paraneoplastic syndromes

a.   Small cell lung cancer.   e.   Neuroendocrine tumour.

b.   Insulinoma.   f.   Gastrinoma.

c.   Phaeochromocytoma.   g.   Germ cell tumour.

d.   Breast cancer.   h.   Brain tumour.

Match the description of the patient's symptoms with the cancer most likely to be causing it.

11) A 50-year-old female presents with central obesity, hirsutism, acne and muscle weakness.

12) A 40-year-old male presents with flushing, diarrhoea, fever and abdominal pain.

13) A 65-year-old male presents to the emergency department with confusion and reduced conscious level. He has a seizure whilst in the department. Bloods show serum sodium to be 112mmol/L and the urinary sodium is high.

14) A 40-year-old female presents with headaches, palpitations and a bilateral fine tremor. She is noted to be hypertensive with a systolic blood pressure of 180mmHg.

15) A 55-year-old male presents to his primary care doctor complaining of the development of prominent breast tissue.

Managing cancer complications

a. Stereotactic radiosurgery.
b. Co-amoxiclav.
c. Chest drain.
d. IV fluids and bisphosphonates.

e. Broad-spectrum antibiotics.
f. Dexamethasone.
g. Radiotherapy.
h. Stenting procedure.

Match the appropriate treatment with the complication of each cancer.

16) A 67-year-old female presents with right-sided weakness and expressive dysphasia. She is known to have breast cancer with lung and bone metastases.

17) A 62-year-old male presents with a history of increasing breathlessness over the last week. A chest radiograph shows a unilateral 'white out' of the lung, and the trachea is deviated away from this.

18) A 55-year-old patient presents to the emergency department pyrexial with a temperature of 39°C, just 3 weeks after completing chemotherapy for tonsillar cancer.

19) A 75-year-old female with melanoma complains of right upper quadrant pain; she is tender in the same area. She is thought to have liver capsule pain.

20) An 82-year-old male presents with delirium, polyuria, low mood and abdominal pain. He has known locally advanced prostate cancer.

Treating cancer

a. Radical.   e. Brachytherapy.

b. Adjuvant.   f. Phase 1 clinical trial.

c. Neoadjuvant.   g. Phase 2 clinical trial.

d. Palliative.   h. Phase 3 clinical trial.

Which of the above terms best describes each definition?

21) Treatment given after surgery to increase the chances of cure.

22) A sealed radiation source is placed next to an area requiring radiotherapy — used most commonly for the treatment of cervical cancer.

23) Treatment that aims for cure of the disease.

24) Comparing a new treatment or treatment regimen to the previously standardised treatment.

25) Testing the initial safety of a new treatment in humans.

Complications of chemotherapy

a.	Neutropenic sepsis.	e.	Tumour lysis syndrome.
b.	Extravasation injury.	f.	Coronary spasm.
c.	Pulmonary embolism.	g.	Palmar plantar syndrome.
d.	Acute kidney injury.	h.	Symptomatic anaemia.

Match the description of the patient with the most likely diagnosis.

26) A 37-year-old female having adjuvant chemotherapy for breast cancer is admitted with a pyrexia 8 days after treatment. She is hypotensive and has a capillary refill time of 5 seconds; her temperature is 38°C.

27) A patient has chest pain whilst receiving an infusion of 5-fluorouracil chemotherapy.

28) During a chemotherapy infusion a patient complains of pain in her hand; the cannula appears to have tissued.

29) An 85-year-old female complains of lethargy, increasing breathlessness on exertion and also occasional chest pain on exertion. She appears pale. She has a known renal cell carcinoma and has had immunotherapy treatment for this.

30) A young patient with ALL is treated with chemotherapy. In the days following chemotherapy, his renal function deteriorates significantly. He is tired and vomits frequently.

Risk factors for cancer

a.	Schistosomiasis infection.	e.	Barrett's oesophagus.
b.	Asbestos exposure.	f.	Late menopause.
c.	HPV 18 exposure.	g.	Multiparity.
d.	*H. pylori* infection.	h.	HRT.

Match the appropriate risk factor for each of the following statements.

31) Protective against ovarian cancer.

32) Associated with bladder cancer.

33) Associated with the development of oesophageal cancer.

34) Associated with gastric cancer.

35) Associated with endometrial cancer.

National cancer screening in the UK

a.	Aged 50-75 years old.	e.	Every 3 years.
b.	Aged 50-64 years old.	f.	Every 5 years.
c.	Aged 60-74 years old.	g.	Colposcopy.
d.	Every 2 years.	h.	Triple assessment.

Match the appropriate screening with each case presented below.

36) Cervical screening for patients aged 25-49 years takes place how often?

37) Breast cancer screening in the 50-70-year age group takes place how often?

38) For which age band does cervical cancer screening change to every 5 years?

39) High-grade cervical intraepithelial neoplasia should be investigated how?

40) What age group is screened for bowel cancer every 2 years?

Inherited cancers

a.	Medullary thyroid carcinoma.	e.	Colorectal cancer.
b.	Leukaemia.	f.	Breast cancer.
c.	Prostate cancer.	g.	Glioma.
d.	Phaeochromocytoma.	h.	Pituitary adenoma.

Which of the above cancers are associated with each of these recognised syndromes or conditions?

41) Multiple endocrine neoplasia Type 1.

42) Von Hippel-Lindau disease.

43) Familial adenomatosis polyposis.

44) Li-Fraumeni syndrome.

45) Peutz-Jeghers syndrome.

Short answer questions

1) A 62-year-old female attends the medical admission unit with a fever. She received a course of adjuvant chemotherapy 2 weeks ago. On examination, she has a temperature of 38.4°C, tachycardia and is hypotensive. She has had a Hickman line *in situ* for the past 2 months. A full blood count shows a white cell count of 1.0×10^4 cells/mm^3.

a. Define sepsis.   2 marks

b. Specify the Sepsis Six.   3 marks

c. What four initial investigations are indicated?   2 marks

d. Name one treatment that should be given immediately.   1 mark

e. If cultures were positive from the Hickman line, what is the definitive   2 marks
    treatment?

2) A 52-year-old male attends the emergency department as he has had 7 days of profuse watery stools. He is currently being treated with pembrolizumab for his locally advanced non-small cell lung cancer. He has been passing watery motions 10-15 times a day, with no blood. He complains of weakness, muscle cramps and paraesthesia. His abdomen is soft and he is tender. He is tachycardic, and his capillary refill time is 5 seconds.

a. Name two organisms that stool screening should investigate.   2 marks

b. Name one imaging investigation that may aid diagnosis.   1 mark

c. If imaging shows a pancolitis, what is the likely cause of his diarrhoea   2 marks
    if microbiological tests were negative?

d. Name three electrolyte abnormalities seen in chronic diarrhoea.   3 marks

e. Give two treatment options for this patient.   2 marks

3) A 75-year-old male presents to his primary care doctor with blood in the urine. He is treated for a UTI but is also referred for further review. Cystoscopy shows evidence of bladder cancer and a CT urogram shows that this is muscle invasive with no metastasis. He is admitted to the ward for new-onset acute kidney injury.

a. What is the most common histology of bladder cancer?   2 marks

b. Name three risk factors for bladder cancer.   3 marks

c. What is the initial surgical management of his malignancy?   1 mark

d. Specify two ward-based treatment options for this patient.   2 marks

e. Name two procedures that may resolve the patient's AKI.   2 marks

4) A 60-year-old female is referred from her primary care doctor with a sore on the roof of her mouth which is painful and non-healing. Further investigations find it to be cancerous but it has not metastasised. The consultant who reviews the patient in clinic recommends radical treatment.

a. Name three risk factors for head and neck cancers.   3 marks

b. What is the likely histological diagnosis of this cancer?   1 mark

c. What is radical therapy and what treatment may be offered?   3 marks
    The same patient develops a sore mouth, odynophagia, trismus and loss of taste. She has visible ulcers in her mouth and a mucous discharge. She has been struggling significantly with poor appetite and a difficulty in eating.

d. What is the diagnosis?   1 mark

e. State two treatments that may help with symptoms.   2 marks

5) An 80-year-old male presents with lower back pain for the last 2 months. He has developed bilateral leg weakness, acute lower abdominal pain and is unable to pass urine. A bladder scan shows 2L of fluid in the bladder and a CT scan shows evidence of metastatic prostate cancer.

a. List four red flag symptoms for back pain. 2 marks
b. What is the most likely diagnosis? 2 marks
c. What imaging would prove the diagnosis, and how would you treat 2 marks
this patient?
d. Biochemically, how is prostate cancer monitored? Histologically, how 2 marks
can prostate cancer be graded?
e. What treatment would be offered given the nature of his disease? 2 marks

6) A 65-year-old female attends the outpatient oncology clinic for consideration of chemotherapy for lung cancer. She has a confirmed right upper lobe mass with evidence of metastases. At present she mobilises with a stick and develops mild breathlessness on exertion. She is able to attend her job in an office and do the housework.

a. Describe the two broad histological classifications of lung cancer. 2 marks
b. Name the system used to grade fitness for chemotherapy. 1 mark
c. What would be this patient's classification? 2 marks
d. Name three antiemetics and describe their mechanism of action. 3 marks
e. The serum sodium is found to be 116mmol/L. Give two possible 2 marks
causes of the hyponatraemia.

7) In the UK all females over the age of 25 years old should be offered screening for cervical cancer. In the UK this takes the form of a cervical smear and HPV testing at various intervals.

a. Name two other cancers which are routinely screened for in the UK.   1 mark

b. Describe three WHO criteria for successful screening programmes.   3 marks

c. Define the following: 4 marks
   i. specificity;
   ii. sensitivity;
   iii. lead time bias;
   iv. length time bias.

d. Which HPV strains predispose to cervical cancer development?   1 mark

e. What staging system is used for cervical cancer?   1 mark

8) A 55-year-old ex-smoker with known small cell cancer presents to the emergency department with symptoms and signs consistent with superior vena cava obstruction.

a. Name three symptoms of superior vena cava obstruction.   3 marks

b. Name two signs of superior vena cava obstruction.   2 marks

c. What imaging would confirm superior vena cava obstruction?   1 mark

d. Specify one medication that should be commenced.   2 marks

e. State two other treatments that can be used to manage a superior vena cava obstruction.   2 marks

9) A 47-year-old female presents to her primary care doctor reporting a palpable lump in her right breast. On examination, it is hard and irregular. She is referred to the breast clinic for triple assessment. She undergoes a lumpectomy and is commenced on Tamoxifen treatment. Routine bloods note a calcium of 3.2mmol/L.

a. Give four common symptoms of breast cancer. 2 marks
b. Specify the three areas of triple assessment for a breast lump. 3 marks
c. What staging system is used to describe breast cancer? 1 mark
d. Give four symptoms of hypercalcaemia. 2 marks
e. Give two medications used to treat hypercalcaemia. 2 marks

10) Radiation therapy delivers energy to tissues resulting in apoptosis of cells and damage to proteins and membranes. It can be used to manage cancer in the curative and palliative setting.

a. Give two types of radiation therapy used in cancer treatment. 2 marks
b. What word is used to describe one session of radiotherapy? 1 mark
c. Name four acute side effects of radiotherapy. 4 marks
d. Name two methods used to ensure a patient's positioning is the same for each session of radiotherapy. 1 mark
e. Name two palliative uses of radiotherapy. 2 marks

11) A 75-year-old female with advanced ovarian cancer and peritoneal metastases had a debulking procedure and is receiving palliative chemotherapy. She presents with a distended and tense abdomen, which is causing discomfort, nausea, a difficulty eating and breathlessness.

a. Describe why ovarian cancer is often detected late. 2 marks
b. Name one marker used to risk stratify for ovarian cancer. 1 mark
c. Describe the WHO analgesic ladder and one example of each level. 3 marks
d. What procedure will improve her symptoms? 2 marks
e. What four common drugs can be given subcutaneously to manage the symptoms experienced at the end of life? 2 marks

12) A 72-year-old male presents with an irregular looking mole on his back. It has been present for several months and he is concerned that it is cancer. His primary care doctor refers him via the 2-week wait pathway.

a.   Name two skin conditions which are considered premalignant for the   2 marks
     development of squamous cell carcinoma of the skin.
b.   What criteria is used in the diagnosis of malignant melanoma?   3 marks
     Describe each feature highlighted by this criteria.
c.   Name three risk factors for the development of melanoma.   3 marks
d.   What curative treatment will be offered if appropriate?   1 mark
e.   What treatment has changed palliative melanoma management?   1 mark

13) A 56-year-old male has a CT scan of his abdomen and pelvis and is found to have pancreatic cancer. He is told the prognosis is very poor.

a.   Why is the prognosis for pancreatic cancer so poor?   2 marks
b.   Describe Courvoisier's law.   2 marks
c.   What staging system is used to describe pancreatic cancer?   1 mark
d.   Describe the pain described by those with pancreatic cancer.   3 marks
e.   State two clinical signs on examination for pancreatic cancer.   2 marks

Chapter 4

Ophthalmology
QUESTIONS

Single best answer questions

1) There are many ophthalmic features to systemic disease; a band-shaped keratopathy is associated with the deposition of which of the following?

a. Calcium.
b. Phosphate.
c. Copper.
d. Iron.

2) A complete third cranial nerve palsy would cause the affected eye to lie in which position?

a. Upwards.
b. Downwards.
c. Upwards and in.
d. Downwards and out.

3) A 50-year-old male presents to the emergency department with visual changes. On examination of his visual field, he has a homonymous hemianopia. Where is the pathology most likely located?

a. Optic chiasm.
b. Optic tract.
c. Optic nerve.
d. Optic radiation.

4) A 58-year-old male with hypertension presents to the emergency department with a sudden loss of vision in his right eye which is painless. On examination, he is found to have an irregular pulse and fundoscopy reveals a bright red appearance of the fovea centralis and retinal whitening. What is the most likely diagnosis?

a. Migraine.
b. Central retinal artery occlusion.
c. Central retinal vein occlusion.
d. Retinal detachment.

5) Which of the following will not be seen in vitamin A deficiency?

a. Night blindness.
b. Bitot's spots.
c. Xerophthalmia.
d. Watery eyes.

6) A 45-year-old male undergoes a series of investigations by his ophthalmologist to investigate the cause of his red eyes. He is found to have a positive Schirmer's test. What is the underlying diagnosis?

a. Dry eyes.
b. Watery eyes.
c. Vitamin D deficiency.
d. Horner's syndrome.

7) A 67-year-old female is admitted to the emergency department with sudden loss of vision; imaging confirms the diagnosis of a right occipital stroke. What visual field defect would this lady present with?

a. Left homonymous hemianopia.
b. Right homonymous hemianopia with macular sparing.
c. Left homonymous hemianopia with macular sparing.
d. Bitemporal hemianopia.

8) A 67-year-old male is diagnosed with glaucoma; the consultant decides to start him on timolol eye drops. How does this class of drug act to reduce the ocular pressure?

a. Increases aqueous outflow via trabecular meshwork.
b. Decreases aqueous humour production by the ciliary body.
c. Increases uveoscleral outflow.
d. Stabilises mast cells.

9) A 34-year-old attends the emergency department with a red right eye, blurred vision and light sensitivity; she has had a feeling of having something in her eye for 24 hours. On examination using fluorescein dye, a linear branching corneal ulcer is found. Which organism most likely causes this finding?

a. *Chlamydia trachomatis.*
b. Herpes simplex virus Type 1.
c. Cytomegalovirus.
d. *Haemophilus influenzae.*

10) The superior rectus acts to move the eye in which direction?

a. Elevation, abduction, inward rotation.
b. Depression, abduction, inward rotation.
c. Elevation, adduction, inward rotation.
d. Depression, adduction, outward rotation.

11) A 26-year-old female attends the emergency department with a sudden loss of vision in the right upper quadrant of her eye; she noticed flashes of light and floaters in her vision. Examination reveals a retinal detachment. Which of the following is a risk factor for this condition?

a. Abdominal surgery.
b. Myopia.
c. Male.
d. Hypotension.

12) A 34-year-old female is seen in the ophthalmology clinic for follow-up and assessment of her long-term health condition. She is found to have a cataract and the ophthalmologist describes it as having a green central disc with spoke-like projections like a sunflower. What is the patient's underlying chronic disease?

a.   Wilson's disease.
b.   Diabetes mellitus.
c.   Chronic alcohol consumption.
d.   Addison's disease.

13) What is the earliest feature that can be seen in anterior uveitis?

a.   Visual loss.
b.   Increased tearing.
c.   Red eye.
d.   Aqueous flare.

14) An 80-year-old male presents with a sudden painless loss of vision. He has scalp tenderness and the blood results reveal a raised ESR and CRP. He undergoes a temporal artery biopsy which confirms the diagnosis of giant cell arteritis. Which condition is associated with this condition?

a.   Hypertension.
b.   Diabetes mellitus.
c.   Polymyalgia rheumatica.
d.   Fibromyalgia.

15) A 45-year-old male has noted drooping to his right eyelid. His pupils react normally to light but his left pupil is larger than the right and he has noticed loss of sweating on the right-hand side of his face. What is the underlying diagnosis?

a. Syphilis.
b. Horner's syndrome.
c. Open angle glaucoma.
d. Third cranial nerve palsy.

16) A 55-year-old male presents to his primary care doctor with a complete third cranial nerve palsy. Which of the following features would not be seen?

a. Ptosis.
b. Diplopia.
c. Down and outward eye position.
d. Miosis.

17) A 54-year-old male presents to the emergency department with a red and painful right eye. The pain started whilst at home reading and has worsened, and he is now vomiting. He has a reduced visual acuity in the right eye and it does not react to light. The right eye is normal. What is the diagnosis?

a. Acute closed angle glaucoma.
b. Scleritis.
c. Blepharitis.
d. Conjunctivitis.

18) A 2-year-old male is seen in the ophthalmology clinic as his father is worried he has a cross-eyed appearance. On examination, he has broad folds of skin covering each eye. The corneal reflex test shows the light to be symmetrical in each eye. A cover test does not show any abnormalities. What is the most likely diagnosis?

a.   Exotropia.
b.   Esotropia.
c.   Pseudostrabismus.
d.   Amblyopia.

19) The inferior oblique acts to move the eye in which direction?

a.   Downwards, abduction, outward rotation.
b.   Downwards, adduction, outward rotation.
c.   Downwards, abduction, inward rotation.
d.   Upwards, adduction, inward rotation.

20) A 20-year-old male presents to his primary care doctor with a 2-day history of a painful red right eye. He has noticed a mucous discharge for the past 24 hours and believes his eye is sticking together. On further questioning, he reveals he has dysuria and pain in his left knee. On examination, he has injected conjunctiva on the right but it is otherwise normal. What is the most likely diagnosis?

a.   Conjunctivitis.
b.   Reiter's syndrome.
c.   Uveitis.
d.   Lyme disease.

21) A 20-year-old male presents to his primary care doctor with a 2-day history of a painful, red, right eye. He has noticed a mucous discharge for the past 24 hours and believes his eye is sticking together. On further questioning, he reveals he has dysuria and pain in his left knee. On examination, he has injected conjunctiva on the right but it is otherwise normal. Which organism is most likely to have caused this patient's symptoms?

a. *Staphylococcus.*
b. *Streptococcus.*
c. *Chlamydia trachomatis.*
d. *Candida albicans.*

22) A 45-year-old male attends his primary care doctor with a 3-day history of a red eye. He states it is very sticky, his eyes feel stuck together and there is something in his eye. On examination, a purulent discharge is seen and diffusely injected conjunctiva. What is the most appropriate treatment?

a. Timolol.
b. Acyclovir.
c. Chlorphenamine.
d. Chloramphenicol.

23) A 16-month-old child is seen in the ophthalmology clinic as his father is worried that he has a cross-eyed appearance. The child's father is concerned as his brother had a similar appearance and had an eye removed due to this problem. On examination, a divergent squint is noted and an absent red reflex. What is the most likely diagnosis?

a. Retinitis pigmentosa.
b. Retinoblastoma.
c. Retinopathy of prematurity.
d. Cataract.

Extended matching questions

Neuro-ophthalmology — pupils

a. Parinaud's syndrome.

b. Argyll-Robertson pupil.

c. Opioid overdose.

d. Third nerve palsy.

e. Adie pupil.

f. Relative afferent pupillary defect.

g. Left Horner's syndrome.

h. Right Horner's syndrome.

Match the description of each of these patient's pupils with the most likely diagnosis.

1) A 23-year-old male presents to his primary care doctor as his friends have noticed he has a dilated pupil that fails to react to light or accommodation.

2) A 57-year-old male presents to the emergency department as he has noticed that his pupils have been irregular for the past 2 days. On examination, he has a semi-dilated pupil that reacts slowly to direct light and accommodation, and is slow to redilate.

3) A 45-year-old female presents to her primary care doctor with a 2-week history of left miosis, facial flushing, anhidrosis and a left drooping eyelid.

4) A 26-year-old female is seen in the neurology clinic following weakness which increases when in the shower. On examination, when a torch light is directed at her right eye, it causes mild constriction of both pupils whilst shining a torch in the left eye causes normal constriction of both pupils.

5) A 28-year-old male is found at home by an ambulance crew unconscious. Neurological examination reveals bilateral small and irregular pupils that are slow to dilate.

Drugs used in ophthalmology

a. Beta-blockers.

b. Prostaglandin analogues.

c. Acetazolamide.

d. Cromoglicate.

e. Hypromellose.

f. Fluorescein.

g. Phenylephrine.

h. Tropicamide.

Match the mechanism of action to the correct drug.

6) Acts to stabilise mast cells to act as an anti-inflammatory agent.

7) Selective alpha-1 adrenergic receptor agonist that acts to dilate pupillary muscles.

8) Used in the treatment of glaucoma by increasing uveoscleral outflow.

9) Used in the identification of corneal ulcers.

10) Used in the treatment of dry eyes to provide artificial tears.

Orbital pathology

a.	Basal cell carcinoma.	e.	Orbital apex syndrome.
b.	Melanoma.	f.	Chalazion.
c.	Orbital fracture.	g.	Squamous cell carcinoma.
d.	Orbital cellulitis.	h.	Dermoid cyst.

Match the description of the patient with the most likely diagnosis.

11) A 50-year-old male attends the ophthalmology clinic with a 16-week history of a nodular lesion on his lower eyelid which has been slowly increasing in size. On examination, a well-defined pearly lesion is noted with a fine network of blood vessels.

12) A 20-year-old male presents to his primary care doctor with an inflamed and mildly painful left eyelid. He has noted a heaviness to his eyelids and increased tearing. On examination, a 1cm nodule is felt on his eyelid but it is not red or warm to the touch.

13) A 45-year-old male attends the ophthalmology clinic with a 2-week history of lid ptosis, changes to his vision with numbness around his upper eyelid and forehead. On examination, he is noted to have ptosis alongside proptosis. He has a fixed and dilated right pupil with complete blindness in his right eye.

14) A 5-year-old male attends his primary care doctor with a 3-day history of a red and swollen eyelid. On examination, he has right-sided swelling with erythema and is warm to the touch. Eye movements are painful and he is noted to have a temperature of 38.4°C.

15) An 80-year-old female presents to the ophthalmology clinic with a 2-month history of a lesion on the left lower eyelid with some mild blurring of vision. The lesion is nodular with dark pigmentation; biopsy notes the presence of atypical melanocytes invading the dermis only.

Visual field defects

a. Right homonymous hemianopia.
b. Right inferior homonymous quadrantanopia.
c. Right homonymous hemianopia with macular sparing.
d. Right central scotoma.
e. Left central scotoma.
f. Bitemporal hemianopia.
g. Left homonymous hemianopia.
h. Left homonymous hemianopia.

Match the description of the patient with the most likely visual field defect.

16) A 58-year-old female is admitted to the stroke unit following a right occipital stroke. Her family are concerned that her vision has changed following the stroke.

17) A 60-year-old male presents to the emergency department with a sudden onset loss of vision. MRI imaging notes a left parietal lobe stroke.

18) A 65-year-old male is diagnosed with an aneurysm following changes in vision associated with a lesion in the right optic tract.

19) A 25-year-old male recently diagnosed with multiple sclerosis is seen by his ophthalmologist to assess his visual field due to changes over the past 4 weeks in his right eye.

20) A 45-year-old female notes a gradual change in vision and headache. She is known to have multiple endocrine neoplasia Type 1 and imaging shows a pituitary adenoma.

Infectious disease and ophthalmology

a.	Candidiasis.	e.	Varicella zoster virus.
b.	Tuberculosis.	f.	Cytomegalovirus.
c.	Toxocariasis.	g.	Rubella.
d.	Syphilis.	h.	Toxoplasmosis.

Match the description of the patient with the most likely diagnosis.

21) A 21-year-old traveller is diagnosed with uveitis on returning from a 3-month trip to Asia. He noted a cough, fever and weight loss whilst travelling and eye issues for 2 weeks. Examination notes cellular aggregates in the anterior segment of the vitreous humor with choroidal granulomas.

22) A 60-year-old male attends his primary care doctor with a 1-month history of visual changes and weakness. Pupillary examination notes small irregular pupils which are unequal and do not respond to light but have a brisk accommodation reflex.

23) A 1-month-old baby is found to have sensorineural deafness, pulmonary artery stenosis and further investigations note retinopathy, cataracts and microphthalmia.

24) A 50-year-old female presents to her primary care doctor with an intense burning redness in her eye. She has blurry vision and is sensitive to light. A blistering rash in noted on her forehead.

25) A 6-year-old is seen following a progressive reduction in vision over 2 days. Vision was initially blurry in the left eye and she now complains of discomfort, redness and pain. Examination reveals a reduced vision acuity on the left. She has a non-reactive left pupil with a hypopyon. She is usually fit and well with two dogs at home.

The red eye

a.	Episcleritis.	e.	Corneal foreign body.
b.	Allergic conjunctivitis.	f.	Dry eye.
c.	Acute closed angle glaucoma.	g.	Endophthalmitis.
d.	Subconjunctival haemorrhage.	h.	Scleritis.

Match the description of the patient with the most likely diagnosis.

26) A 16-year-old attends his primary care doctor with a 2-week history of itchy red eyes with a similar episode 12 months ago. He describes them as feeling sticky. On examination, there is a watery discharge with some mucus. You note a cobblestone appearance of the superior tarsal conjunctiva.

27) A 45-year-old steel worker attends the emergency department with a sudden onset pain in his right eye whilst at work associated with increased lacrimation. On examination, he is keeping his eye held firmly closed and on opening you note it appears intensely red.

28) A 60-year-old female underwent cataract surgery 7 days ago. She presents with a painful red eye. On examination, pus is seen in the anterior chamber and the red reflex is absent.

29) A 40-year-old female presents to the emergency department with a sharp pain in her right eye, reduced visual acuity and vomiting. Examination reveals a red right eye with a fixed mid-dilated pupil, ciliary injection and raised intraocular pressure at 55mmHg. Her left eye is normal.

30) A 26-year-old female with a history of rheumatoid arthritis presents with a sudden onset painful red eye with blurring of vision. Examination notes intense scleral injection and examination is very painful.

Systemic disease and ophthalmology

a.   Diabetes mellitus.   e.   Retinoblastoma.

b.   Neurofibromatosis Type 1.   f.   Intracranial hypertension.

c.   Neurofibromatosis Type 2.   g.   Wilson's disease.

d.   Multiple sclerosis.   h.   Graves' disease.

Match the description of the patient with the most likely diagnosis.

31)   A 20-year-old female is admitted to the emergency department with vomiting, weakness and jaundice. On examination, a brown ring is present around her cornea. On further questioning, she states her uncle had a condition involving his liver and kidneys.

32)   A 25-year-old male attends the emergency department with muscle weakness and blurred vision. He has noted an electrical sensation running down his back when bending his neck. On examination, the topic disc appears pale and swollen.

33)   A 5-year-old male is seen in the ophthalmology clinic for proptosis. Examination reveal multiple nodules that are brown and gelatinous in nature on the iris and MRI notes an optic nerve glioma.

34)   A 3-year-old male is brought to her primary care doctor following her family noticing that her left eye appears white in recent photographs. On examination, the red reflex on the left is absent. Fundoscopy reveals a cream-coloured mass with increased vascularisation.

35)   A 55-year-old female sees her primary care doctor for proptosis and double vision. She has a lid retraction, lid lag and exophthalmos. You also note a fine tremor in her hands.

Sudden visual loss

a. Central retinal artery occlusion.
b. Giant cell arteritis.
c. Central retinal vein occlusion.
d. Retinal detachment.

e. Diabetic maculopathy.
f. Migraine.
g. Pituitary tumour.
h. Optic neuritis.

Match the description of the patient with the most likely diagnosis.

36) A 60-year-old male attends the emergency department with a sudden loss of vision, headache and pain in his jaw. On examination, he has scalp tenderness and blood tests reveal a raised ESR.

37) A 65-year-old male with a history of hypertension and a previous CABG presents with sudden loss of vision in his right eye. He denies any pain. His left eye is normal. Fundoscopy shows a central red retinal area surrounded by pale areas.

38) A 21-year-old female attends the emergency department following a sudden loss of vision bilaterally, headaches, nausea and bright lights in her vision. On assessment, all symptoms have resolved.

39) A 40-year-old female with a history of myopia attends the eye casualty with a sudden flash of light in the upper corner of her vision which has lasted for the past 8 hours. She has noted a headache and floaters in her left eye but denies any pain, tearing or loss of vision.

40) A 20-year-old male presents to his primary care doctor with a sudden loss of vision in his left eye over the past 2 days. He has pain when looking left and visual acuity is reduced in his left eye. Examination reveals a swollen optic disc. He has noticed his vision is worsened in a hot shower.

Gradual loss of vision

a.   Open angle glaucoma.

b.   Diabetic maculopathy.

c.   Occipital tumour.

d.   Retinitis pigmentosa.

e.   Uncorrected refractive error.

f.   Optic nerve tumour.

g.   Cataract.

h.   Pituitary tumour.

Match the description of the patient with the most likely diagnosis.

41)   A 50-year-old with hypertension attends an optician for regular review. On assessment, a raised intraocular pressure at 28mmHg is detected; vision is not affected and pupils are normal.

42)   A 72-year-old female attends her primary care doctor for a gradual loss of vision. She has increasing difficulty seeing out of her right eye and no longer drives at night due to seeing halos around lights. On examination, eye movements are normal in both eyes but the red reflex is absent on the right.

43)   A 60-year-old Type 2 diabetic has a routine retinal screening. He has noted a decrease in central vision and previous screenings have noted background diabetic retinopathy.

44)   A 26-year-old female presents to her primary care doctor with a gradual loss of vision. On examination, there is a symmetrical loss in the outer half of the right and left visual fields.

45)   A 14-year-old attends his primary care doctor with his mother as he can no longer see the whiteboard from his seat in class. He is usually fit and well. Visual acuity is 6/12. All other examinations are normal.

Short answer questions

1) A 65-year-old male attends the emergency department with a sharp pain in his left eye, reduced visual acuity and vomiting. Examination reveals a red left eye with a fixed mid-dilated pupil, ciliary injection and raised intraocular pressure at 55mmHg. His right eye is normal.

a. What is the underlying diagnosis?   1 mark

b. Name two anatomical risk factors for developing this condition.   2 marks

c. What is the underlying mechanism of this condition?   2 marks

d. Describe one supportive measure and two drugs to acutely reduce ocular pressure.   3 marks

e. State two measures that may be taken once the acute attack has resolved.   2 marks

2) A 6-year-old male attends the primary care doctor surgery with bilaterally red, itchy eyes that started 4 days ago; it initially started in his right eye but now both of his eyes are affected. He says his eyes are sticky and feel gritty. On examination, you note bilateral mild chemosis, a purulent discharge and you suspect bacterial conjunctivitis.

a. Define three other common causes of an acute red eye.   3 marks

b. Name two causative organisms of this condition in this age group.   2 marks

c. Specify one treatment and two pieces of advice you would offer.   2 marks

d. Identify two differences for a patient with allergic conjunctivitis.   1 mark

e. If the patient was a neonate with a mother treated for sexually transmitted disease during pregnancy what bacterial organisms should be considered and what would be the most appropriate treatment for each?   2 marks

3) A 74-year-old female attends the ophthalmology clinic with a 2-year progressive loss of vision in her left eye. She feels well in herself with no other past medical history. She has found it more difficult to drive at night as she experiences glare from oncoming vehicles and on examination, you note a decreased visual acuity and an absent red reflex on the left.

a. What is the underlying diagnosis?   1 mark
b. Name three common ocular risk factors for this condition.   3 marks
c. State two categories this condition is divided into based on age of   2 marks
    onset.
d. What surgical treatment can be offered to this patient?   1 mark
e. What is the complication that can occur within 7 days of surgery   3 marks
    which requires urgent management to prevent loss of vision and
    name two methods to treat this condition?

4) A 67-year-old female attends her primary care doctor with a 3-day history of a mild intermittent tingling sensation over her forehead. She has noticed a rash has started to form in the same region and on the tip of her nose which feels like a burning and itchy sensation. She has no past medical history.

a. What is the diagnosis and causative organism?   2 marks
b. The rash extending to the tip of her nose is known as Hutchinson's   2 marks
    sign — why is this an important examination finding?
c. Which dermatome is usually affected in this condition?   1 mark
d. What treatment would be offered for this patient and how would this   2 marks
    differ for an immunosuppressed patient?
e. What complication may result as a consequence of this infection and   3 marks
    what two treatments could be offered?

5) A 24-year-old with known rheumatoid arthritis presents to his primary care doctor with a 4-day history of severe pain in his right eye which he describes as a deep pain. He has noticed blurring of vision and photophobia. On examination, his right eye is a deep red which does not resolve on gentle pressure to the conjunctiva and performing this is exquisitely tender. You suspect this patient has anterior scleritis.

a. Name four other risk factors for this condition. 2 marks

b. State two other findings on examination in this condition. 2 marks

c. Describe two actions that should be performed if scleritis is suspected. 2 marks

d. List four ways scleritis differs from episcleritis. 2 marks

e. Name two treatments for episcleritis. 2 marks

6) A 6-year-old male attends the emergency department with his mother following a 4-day history of a red and swollen eyelid. On examination, he has left-sided swelling with erythema that is warm to the touch. Eye movements are painful and he is noted to have a temperature of 38.4°C.

a. What is the underlying diagnosis? 1 mark

b. Name two organisms responsible for this condition. 2 marks

c. State two risk factors for this condition. 2 marks

d. What treatment should be commenced and where should this condition be managed? 2 marks

e. What other orbital inflammatory condition should this diagnosis be differentiated from and name four differences in how these conditions will present? 3 marks

7) A 25-year-old medical student is preparing for final year examinations. She is practising cranial nerve examination with a friend and she is unable to move her left eye laterally.

a. Which cranial nerve has been affected in this patient? 2 marks
b. Which muscle is supplied by this nerve and what is its function? 1 mark
c. Name two other features you would expect to see on examination. 2 marks
d. List six potential causes of this patient's pathology in adults. 3 marks
e. Specify two medical treatment options for this patient. 2 marks

8) A 64-year-old female with hypertension presents to the emergency department with a sudden painless loss of vision in her left eye. Fundoscopy reveals a bright red appearance of the fovea centralis and retinal whitening. The doctor thinks that this is a cherry spot appearance of the retina and diagnoses central retinal artery occlusion.

a. Name four associated diseases for this condition. 2 marks
b. What is the most common cause of retinal artery occlusion? 1 mark
c. Specify two other possible findings on examination. 2 marks
d. Name three investigations for this condition. 3 marks
e. Define two differences between a central retinal artery occlusion and 2 marks
a branch occlusion.

9) A 65-year-old male attends the ophthalmology clinic following a recent review by his primary care doctor in which his blood pressure was found to be 165/100mmHg with several changes on fundoscopy indicating Grade 3 hypertensive retinopathy. He has a past medical history of Type 2 diabetes mellitus and chronic kidney disease.

a.   Name four other modifiable risk factors for hypertension.   2 marks

b.   Name four changes seen in Grade 3 hypertensive retinopathy.   2 marks

c.   What is the target blood pressure for this patient?   1 mark

d.   Name two other ophthalmic complications of hypertension.   1 mark

e.   Name four groups of commonly used antihypertensives.   4 marks

10) A 56-year-old Type 2 diabetic female attends her primary care doctor for a regular diabetic review. As part of the examination, the doctor examines her eyes and notes the presence of cotton wool spots, exudate, with dot and blot haemorrhages which were not present 1 year ago.

a.   What is the underlying diagnosis?   2 marks

b.   If this condition was more advanced, name three additional   3 marks
     ophthalmic findings.

c.   Name two conditions that give a similar retinal appearance to this   2 marks
     condition.

d.   If the patient reported loss of central vision in addition to the above   1 mark
     symptoms, what condition would you suspect?

e.   Name two methods to reduce progression of this condition at an   2 marks
     early stage.

11) A 72-year-old male is seen in the ophthalmology clinic following a gradual loss of vision in his right eye and vision is blurred. He finds it hard to recognise faces, drive or read. He is diagnosed with age-related macular degeneration (ARMD).

a.   What visual area is classically affected in ARMD?   1 mark

b.   How is this condition classified and define each type?   3 marks

c.   Define the pathology behind each type of ARMD.   2 marks

d.   Name four risk factors for this condition.   2 marks

e.   Name four management options for this patient.   2 marks

12) A 4-year-old female is brought to her primary care doctor following her family noticing that her right eye appears white in recent photographs. On examination, the red reflex on the right is absent. Her mother believes that her brother had a similar condition as a child in which he had to have his eye removed. Fundoscopy reveals a cream-coloured mass with increased vascularisation.

a.	What is the underlying diagnosis?	1 mark
b.	Name three other causes of leukocoria.	3 marks
c.	Specify two investigations for this patient.	2 marks
d.	State two treatment options that should be considered for this patient.	2 marks
e.	List two supportive treatments that could be offered to this patient.	2 marks

13) A 26-year-old male attends the emergency department with a sudden painless loss of vision in his right eye following an altercation in a nightclub. He reports blurred vision and a dark shadow is present on the edge of his vision. Fundoscopy reveals a wrinkled grey area on his retina in keeping with a retinal detachment.

a.	Name the two layers of the retina.	1 marks
b.	Specify the three types of retinal detachment.	3 marks
c.	Name two causes of retinal detachment.	2 marks
d.	State four other symptoms of a retinal detachment other than those described.	2 marks
e.	What two treatment options could be offered to this patient?	2 marks

Chapter 5

Paediatrics
QUESTIONS

Single best answer questions

1) A 2-week-old preterm infant is admitted to the ward following reduced feeding, stomach distention and vomiting blood-stained fluid. The nursing staff noted that his blood pressure has fallen since his initial assessment in the emergency department 1 hour ago and he is tachycardic. What is your first-line investigation?

a. Aspirate vomit.
b. Abdominal X-ray.
c. Blood tests including CRP.
d. Ultrasound abdomen.

2) A new mother wants to discuss her son who was born with Down's syndrome as she does not understand the consequences of this diagnosis. Which of the following is not a feature of Down's syndrome?

a. Congenital heart defects.
b. Brushfield spots.
c. Duodenal atresia.
d. Vascular dementia.

3) An 8-month-old infant is seen by his primary care doctor following parental concerns that he is not developing at the same rate as his siblings. Which of the following should always be attained at this age?

a. Sits with support.
b. Reaches and grasps.
c. Pulls to stand.
d. Can build a tower of three bricks.

4) The mother of a 16-year-old girl has come to ask you about her daughter, who has not yet undergone menarche. She is worried that her daughter is not developing as quickly as other girls. Gonadotrophin levels are low. Which of the following diagnoses best accounts for these findings?

a. Klinefelter's syndrome.
b. Turner's syndrome.
c. Crohn's disease.
d. Androgen insensitivity syndrome.

5) A 2-year-old child is seen by her primary care doctor after moving to the UK from Pakistan. On examination, you find a bowing deformity of her legs and she is small for her age with widening of wrists and ankles. Which of the following would you expect to find if bloods were taken?

a. Low calcium, low vitamin D, high PTH.
b. Low calcium, low vitamin D, low PTH.
c. High calcium, low vitamin D, high PTH.
d. Low calcium, high vitamin D, low PTH.

6) A 3-month-old child presents with paroxysmal episodes of abdominal pain, drawing her legs up and becoming pale. She is refusing feeds and her abdomen is slightly distended. On examination, you feel a sausage-shaped mass in the abdomen and the parents report three episodes of red-coloured stools. Which investigation would confirm the characteristic diagnostic sign for this condition?

a.   Abdominal X-ray.
b.   CT chest, abdomen and pelvis.
c.   MRI abdomen.
d.   Ultrasound abdomen.

7) A 9-month-old presents to the emergency department with a sharp, dry cough and tachypnoea, preceded by coryzal symptoms. On auscultation, you note widespread fine inspiratory crackles and high-pitched expiratory wheezing. What is the most likely causative organism?

a.   Human metapneumovirus.
b.   Parainfluenza virus.
c.   Respiratory syncytial virus.
d.   *Mycoplasma pneumoniae*.

8) Constipation is a common complaint in children and causes parental concern. They can often be reassured, but which of the following would you treat as a red flag in a well child with decreased stool frequency?

a.   Vomiting.
b.   Failure to thrive.
c.   Mild abdominal distension.
d.   Overflow soiling.

9) A breastfed child is seen in clinic following a 10-week history of being persistently distressed after feeding for at least 4 hours per day. He frequently regurgitates feeds, has diarrhoea and develops a rash shortly after feeding. The mother wishes to continue breastfeeding. What should you advise the mother?

a. Stop breastfeeding completely and move to formula feed.
b. A course of antihistamines and continue to feed normally.
c. Eliminate cow's milk protein from his diet and review symptoms.
d. Eliminate lactose from his diet and review symptoms.

10) A 10-year-old boy's parents have come to see you concerned about his short stature. Which of the following does not often present with short stature?

a. Hypothyroidism.
b. Turner syndrome.
c. Noonan syndrome.
d. Klinefelter syndrome.

11) An 11-month-old child has had a persistent facial port-wine stain since birth. This has not resolved and the child has now started having seizures. Which of the following often occurs in this condition?

a. Café au lait patches.
b. Complete deafness.
c. Glaucoma.
d. Peripheral cyanosis.

12) The parents of a 6-year-old child attend his primary care doctor as they are worried he is wetting the bed at night. He previously achieved continence at the age of 3. Which of the following situations would require further investigation?

a.   Children with enuresis secondary to constipation.
b.   Children with enuresis during the day.
c.   Children with isolated nocturnal enuresis.
d.   Children with a history of recurrent UTI.

13) A 3-year-old child is admitted to the paediatric ward for treatment of a lower respiratory tract infection; 2 days into her stay she has a seizure lasting for 5 minutes. The child's temperature at the time of the seizure is 38°C and she recovers quickly without treatment. No previous history of seizures is reported. What is the most likely cause of this episode?

a.   Simple febrile seizure.
b.   Reflex anoxic attack.
c.   Complex febrile seizure.
d.   West syndrome.

14) You are called by the nursing staff to prescribe fluids for a 7-year-old child who weighs 27kg. He is not taking any fluid orally. His height is 128cm. Assuming that he does not need correction for dehydration, what is the rate in ml/hr of fluid that he requires?

a.   68ml/hour.
b.   56ml/hour.
c.   78ml/hour.
d.   136ml/hour.

15) The parents of a 14-year-old girl are worried that she has ADHD; she makes careless mistakes at school (W), she does not listen when she is spoken to directly, she loses things easily, she talks excessively with friends but not at all to adults (X), and at home interrupts her family. She complains of being anxious all the time (Y) and can't stop moving. These symptoms have been present for the last 3 months (Z), following the break-up of her parents. Which of the above features would not suggest a diagnosis of ADHD?

a.   W, X, Y and Z.
b.   X and Y.
c.   Y and Z.
d.   X, Y and Z.

16) A 7-year-old child has developed a rash following a fever; she now has a coarse erythematous rash over her face and scapula with a white strawberry tongue. What is the likely causative organism?

a.   *Staphylococcus aureus*.
b.   Human Herpes virus 6.
c.   *Streptococcus pyogenes*.
d.   *Streptococcus pneumoniae*.

17) A 3-month-old child presents with a 7-day history of coryza followed by coughing and vomiting. The child shows evidence of apnoeic episodes; a nasal swab reveals a *Bordetella* organism. Which of the following is the most likely course of this disease?

a. May persist for many months, complications are uncommon.
b. Resolves quickly, complications are common.
c. Resolves quickly, complications are uncommon.
d. May persist for many months, complications are common.

18) A female in her third trimester comes into contact with chickenpox; 2 days later she delivers her newborn 1 week prematurely. The child is healthy and does not have a rash. What treatment should be given to the infant?

a. None; chickenpox is usually benign and she can be reassured.
b. The neonate should be given immunoglobulin and acyclovir.
c. The neonate should be admitted to a neonatal intensive care unit as death from varicella zoster virus in early life is extremely high.
d. Monitor for signs of rash and treat as in older children if a rash develops.

19) A 9-year-old child develops a progressive neurological deficit over 12 months. He is diagnosed as having subacute sclerosing panencephalitis. Which condition is he likely to have had early in life that led to this?

a. Mumps.
b. Measles.
c. Cytomegalovirus.
d. Varicella zoster virus.

20) A 3-year-old is seen by her primary care doctor following a prolonged fever for 6 days. She is diagnosed with Kawasaki disease and appropriate treatment is commenced. Which of the following is not a major criteria for diagnosing Kawasaki disease?

a. Raised ESR.
b. Polymorphous rash.
c. Erythema of the extremities.
d. A strawberry tongue.

21) A 5-year-old girl presents with pain in her left ear and reduced hearing. On examination, you see a perforation of the left eardrum with otorrhoea, and a non-erythematous canal. What is the most likely diagnosis?

a. Acute otitis media.
b. Otitis externa.
c. Otitis media with effusion.
d. Petrositis.

22) A 7-year-old boy presents with 2-day history of painful swallowing. On examination, he is pyrexial, with a tonsillar exudate, tender cervical lymphadenopathy and no evidence of a cough. You suspect tonsillitis. What should be used to treat this child?

a. No treatment is required as the disease is self-limiting.
b. Amoxicillin.
c. Phenoxymethylpenicillin.
d. Co-amoxiclav.

23) A 3-year-old girl presents to the emergency department with a 2-hour history of a barking cough, stridor and mild dyspnoea. She has a hoarse voice and is declining food but is still drinking fluids. What is the most likely causative organism?

a. Parainfluenza virus.
b. Respiratory syncytial virus.
c. *Haemophilus influenzae*.
d. Human metapneumovirus.

Extended matching questions

Common syndromes

a. Down's syndrome.

b. Edwards syndrome.

c. Fragile X syndrome.

d. Prader-Willi syndrome.

e. Angelman syndrome.

f. Turner syndrome.

g. Cri du chat syndrome.

h. DiGeorge syndrome.

Match the description of the patient with the most likely diagnosis.

1) A 10-year-old girl has crowded teeth, long-term issues with hearing, a short neck and wide-spaced nipples.

2) A 4-year-old boy has a low IQ, a high forehead, large testicles, facial asymmetry and long ears. He has features of autism.

3) An infant has a low birth weight and slow growth with feeding difficulties and persistent inspiratory stridor. Her parents report she has an odd cry.

4) A 3-week-old infant has been floppy since birth and has brachycephaly and speckles in her iris. She has a heart murmur and short little finger.

5) A 5-year-old obese boy with a narrow face, genital hypoplasia and developmental delay. He eats excessively and has frequent tantrums.

Childhood strabismus

a. Esotropia.   e. Esophoria.
b. Exotropia.   f. Exophoria.
c. Hypertropia.   g. Hyperphoria.
d. Hypotropia.   h. Hypophoria.

Match the visual abnormality with the correct description.

6) The visual axis of the affected eye is above that of the fixating eye.

7) A tendency for one or both eyes to drift outward typically when covering the other eye.

8) When both eyes are open, one eye is turned inwards.

9) A tendency of the visual axis of one eye to deviate downward, prevented by binocular vision.

10) The visual axis of the affected eye is below that of the fixating eye.

Acute abdominal pain

a. Mesenteric adenitis.
b. Acute appendicitis.
c. Intussusception.
d. Meckel's diverticulum.

e. Urinary tract infection.
f. Diabetic ketoacidosis.
g. Crohn's disease.
h. Constipation.

Match the description of the patient with the most likely diagnosis.

11) A 5-year-old child attends his primary care doctor as his parents are concerned that he has not eaten for the past 2 days and has been vomiting for the past 6 hours. On examination, he has generalised abdominal tenderness with guarding and a low-grade fever.

12) A 1-year-old child presents to his primary care doctor with recurrent abdominal pain, associated with crying on the toilet and intermittent diarrhoea.

13) A 1-year-old child attends the emergency department with inconsolable crying and drawing her legs towards her abdomen. Her parents are concerned as she has passed a different coloured stool which they describe as redcurrant jelly in appearance.

14) A 6-year-old child presents with weight loss, diarrhoea, abdominal pain and lethargy. A biopsy reveals evidence of non-caseating epithelioid granulomas.

15) A 1-year-old who was previously well presents with an inability to pass stool followed by abdominal pain and vomiting. Earlier in life they had bright red painless rectal bleeding, which settled.

Common skin rashes in children

a. Chickenpox.

b. Eczema.

c. Erythema multiforme.

d. Scarlet fever.

e. Measles.

f. Molluscum contagiosum.

g. Scabies.

h. Parvovirus B19.

Match the description of the patient with the most likely diagnosis.

16) A 4-year-old child is unwell with a fever, followed by a coarse palpable rash 24 hours later. The rash started over the neck and scapula and spread to the trunk and legs. There is an area of pallor around the mouth.

17) A 7-year-old child presents to the primary care doctor with a 7-day history of coryza. She develops an erythematous rash on her face, sparing the nose, which spreads to her extremities.

18) A 2-year-old boy develops a fever and widespread rash comprising of papules, vesicles, pustules and crusty lesions.

19) A 13-year-old develops clusters of firm, smooth umbilicated papules on his trunk and extremities.

20) A 7-year-old presents to her primary care doctor with a dull red urticarial plaque on her right arm which slowly enlarges over 4 days. She has coryzal symptoms.

Jaundice

a.	Physiological jaundice.	e.	Biliary atresia.
b.	Haemolytic disease of the newborn.	f.	Breast milk.
c.	Galactosaemia.	g.	Hypothyroidism.
d.	Alpha-1 antitrypsin deficiency.	h.	G6PD deficiency.

Match the description of the patient with the most likely diagnosis.

21) A term infant of normal weight presents with prolonged jaundice, pale stools and dark urine. Liver function tests show a conjugated hyperbilirubinaemia and high GGT.

22) A term infant presents with jaundice 3 days post-delivery which resolves within 1 week; he remains well throughout this episode.

23) A 6-week-old infant presents with *E. coli* sepsis. On examination, he is jaundiced, has hepatomegaly, cataracts, and a failure to thrive. He is treated and returns home. Later in life he has global developmental delay.

24) A 1-year-old child presents with dysuria and incontinence. The clerking doctor suspects a UTI and treats with nitrofurantoin. Two days later she returns to the emergency department with jaundice. She has a previous history of neonatal jaundice. A blood film shows Heinz bodies.

25) A 28-year-old female who has missed her antenatal visits gives birth to a baby who is unwell early in life, with jaundice, hepatosplenomegaly, oedema, petechiae and ascites.

Failure to thrive

a. Cystic fibrosis.
b. Hypothyroidism.
c. Chronic kidney disease.
d. Asthma.

e. Neglect.
f. Coeliac disease.
g. Fetal alcohol syndrome.
h. Phenylketonuria.

Match the description of the patient with the most likely diagnosis.

26) A 6-month-old infant has feeding difficulties, a low-frequency cry, constipation and jaundice. On examination, he has a large tongue.

27) An infant is born small for dates, with a small head, thin upper lip and microphthalmia. He is constantly hungry, and has a low IQ with speech and language delays.

28) A child had meconium ileus at birth with prolonged jaundice. She develops recurrent chest infections and chronic issues with foul-smelling stools.

29) A child is pale with light blue eyes. The patient has a mousy odour, failure to thrive, and eczematous skin.

30) A child is investigated for a failure to thrive. She smells musty and she has been treated for recurrent scabies infections.

Congenital heart disease

a.   Patent ductus arteriosus.

b.   Patent foramen ovale.

c.   Coarctation of the aorta.

d.   Tetralogy of Fallot

e.   Transposition of the great vessels.

f.   Hypoplastic left heart.

g.   Ventricular septal defect (VSD).

h.   Atrial septal defect (ASD).

Match the description of the patient with the most likely diagnosis.

31)   A 4-year-old child visits his primary care doctor as his mother is concerned regarding his pink appearance. On auscultation, there is obliteration of the second heart sound by a harsh systolic murmur best heard at the left sternal edge.

32)   A 3-year-old child attends his primary care doctor as his mother is concerned regarding his pink appearance. On examination, there is a widely split second heart sound and a soft ejection systolic murmur in the pulmonary area.

33)   An 8-month-old infant is seen in the paediatric clinic following a low birthweight and poor feeding. The child is short of breath and becomes blue after episodes of prolonged crying. On auscultation, there is a systolic murmur with a thrill and an aortic ejection click.

34)   A neonate is initially well, then suddenly becomes unwell and turns blue. On auscultation, there is a systolic murmur in the left infraclavicular area.

35)   A 6-month-old infant has tachypnoea and tachycardia. On auscultation, there is a continuous machinery murmur at the left upper sternal border.

Funny turns and seizures

a. Febrile seizure.

b. Syncope.

c. Reflex anoxic seizure.

d. Night terror.

e. Fabricated illness.

f. Absence seizure.

g. Dravet syndrome.

h. Juvenile myoclonic epilepsy.

What is the most likely cause of each of the following 'funny turns'?

36) A 6-year-old female becomes frightened, going pale and limp. She loses consciousness with a brief period of stiffening and jerking her limbs. She is tired and washed out following the episode.

37) A 16-year-old male attends his primary care doctor with several episodes of early morning sudden jerking motions of his arms and shoulders. He later develops generalised tonic clonic seizures.

38) A previously healthy infant develops severe myoclonic epilepsy with recurrent febrile hemiclonic seizures.

39) A 13-year-old girl is standing in assembly when she collapses suddenly. She has several jerking movements of her arms and legs and is rousable. She quickly knows where she is and feels slightly unwell.

40) An 8-year-old boy has an episode of collapse that he is unable to recall. A teacher in class is unable to get his attention for 20 seconds and he does not seem to be responding, he is then rousable and can talk normally.

Childhood cancers

a. Acute lymphoblastic leukaemia.
b. Acute myeloid leukaemia.
c. Ewing sarcoma.
d. Hodgkin's lymphoma.

e. Neuroblastoma.
f. Wilms' tumour.
g. Non-Hodgkin's lymphoma.
h. Langerhans cell histiocytosis.

Match the description of the patient with the most likely diagnosis.

41) A 10-year-old boy with Down's syndrome develops an acute illness over 3 days. He is fatigued; blood tests reveal anaemia, thrombocytopenia, a high white cell count, neutropenia, blasts and raised LDH.

42) A 4-year-old is investigated for visible haematuria. On examination, he has a unilateral abdominal mass.

43) A 3-year-old girl presents with fatigue and malaise; blood tests reveal anaemia, thrombocytopenia and neutropenia. Bone marrow aspiration shows the presence of significant numbers of blasts and she has a t(9;22)(q34.1;q11.2) translocation.

44) A 15-year-old boy presents with pain in his left arm. On examination, a painful mass is felt and X-ray shows an onion-skin appearance to the lesion.

45) A 12-year-old girl presents with an enlarged lymph node with no other obvious intercurrent illness. A biopsy reveals Reed-Sternberg cells.

Short answer questions

1) A 1-week-old infant appears to be short of breath from birth. The assessing clinician suspects tetralogy of Fallot.

a.	What four features make up tetralogy of Fallot?	4 marks
b.	Give two signs that may be detected on auscultation.	2 marks
c.	State two presenting signs or symptoms of tetralogy of Fallot.	2 marks
d.	What is the most common finding on an ECG?	1 mark
e.	Which other abnormality makes up the pentalogy of Fallot?	1 mark

2) Parents of a 5-day-old infant have requested information regarding the newborn blood spot screening test. The parents would like to know more about this test.

a.	Name three other diseases screened for this test.	3 marks
b.	State two other conditions which are screened for in the UK during the first 6-8 weeks of life.	2 marks
c.	Specify two signs or symptoms of phenylketonuria (PKU).	2 marks
d.	Give two signs or symptoms of neonatal congenital hypothyroidism.	2 marks
e.	What causes PKU?	1 mark

3) At a routine 8-week check, a baby is noted to have an abnormal shape to its pelvis. The primary care doctor refers the baby to the paediatric hip clinic to assess for evidence of hip abnormalities. The orthopaedic surgeon suspects the child may have developmental dysplasia of the hip (DDH).

a. State the two examinations used to assess for DDH in infants and describe each examination. — 4 marks

b. Which investigation is first-line for hip imaging in infants? — 1 mark

c. What would you see on this imaging modality in DDH? — 1 mark

d. Name two complications associated with DDH. — 2 marks

e. Specify two treatments that can be used for DDH. — 2 marks

4) An infant has a difficult and prolonged birth. As the infant begins to develop he exhibits a series of features associated with cerebral palsy.

a. Give three motor features of cerebral palsy. — 3 marks

b. What is the common unifying cause of cerebral palsy? — 1 mark

c. Name three types of cerebral palsy. — 3 marks

d. What is the neonatal scoring system of which a low score indicates that the child is at a higher risk of developing cerebral palsy? — 1 mark

e. Name two treatments for muscle spasms in children. — 2 marks

5) The parents of a 4-month-old infant are concerned regarding reflux. They suspect the symptoms have been present for the past 3 months.

a. Name two symptoms of gastro-oesophageal reflux disease (GORD). — 2 marks

b. Give two risk factors for the development of GORD. — 2 marks

c. State two investigations used in more severe cases of GORD. — 1 mark

d. What is the key difference between reflux and vomiting? — 1 mark

e. Name four red flags in this patient that may prompt you to consider alternative diagnoses to GORD. — 4 marks

6) A 3-month-old infant presents to the emergency department with a 2-week history of vomiting and poor oral intake. Following a thorough history and examination, you suspect pyloric stenosis.

a. Give three features of the vomiting that may lead you to suspect this is pyloric stenosis.   3 marks

b. What can often be felt in the abdomen in pyloric stenosis; where is this normally felt?   2 marks

c. Specify the main diagnostic test for this condition.   1 mark

d. State the initial treatment for pyloric stenosis with persistent vomiting. What treatment is then needed?   2 marks

e. What abnormalities are often seen on a blood gas as a result of this condition?   2 marks

7) The National Institute for Health and Care Excellence (NICE) has produced a traffic light system to be utilised by clinicians to identify paediatric patients at risk of serious illness in order to prompt appropriate management. This system uses a series of clinical features to stratify the risk of severity of an acute disease.

a. State four green features.   2 marks

b. Give four yellow features.   2 marks

c. Name four red features.   2 marks

d. Broadly, what should be done with children in each 'category' by a non-paediatric specialist?   3 marks

e. Define the Sepsis 6.   1 mark

8) An 8-year-old boy with asthma is admitted with shortness of breath and wheeze. He is clearly distressed and you suspect this patient may have a life-threatening asthma exacerbation.

a. Describe the pathophysiology of asthma. 2 marks

b. Give three features for a life-threatening exacerbation of asthma. 3 marks

c. In an 8-year-old child with poorly controlled asthma on salbutamol alone, what is the next step in the treatment protocol? 1 mark

d. What are the three initial treatments that should be urgently given in life-threatening asthma? 3 marks

e. What is status asthmaticus? 1 mark

9) A 7-year-old child presents to the emergency department following a seizure. The parents have noted several seizures over the last 2 months, but these were not previously reported. You suspect that he has epilepsy.

a. What is the definition of epilepsy? 2 marks

b. State the definition of a seizure. 2 marks

c. Give the two main categories (types) of seizures. 1 mark

d. Define SUDEP. 3 marks

e. Name two conditions that may mimic seizures. 2 marks

10) A 5-year-old girl presents with a 10-week history of stiffness in her right knee and left ankle. This is worse in the morning; she complains of mild pain in her legs when she first wakes up. She is otherwise well and no other joints are affected.

a. What is the most likely diagnosis? 2 marks

b. What is the most likely abnormality found in her blood tests? 1 mark

c. Give two other organs commonly affected in this condition. 2 marks

d. Give three pharmacological treatments for this condition. 3 marks

e. Whilst in hospital, you encounter a similar patient with Still's disease. 2 marks
   Other than arthralgia name two major criteria of this disease.

11) A 4-year-old child undergoing treatment for acute lymphoblastic leukaemia is seen on the ward following treatment. She reports feeling unwell and her parents are concerned she is not eating.

a. What is the difference between acute myeloid leukaemia (AML) and 2 marks
   acute lymphoblastic leukaemia (ALL)?

b. Give four clinical features that may be seen in the initial presentation 2 marks
   of this patient.

c. What would you see on a blood film in this patient? 1 mark

d. Give three treatments for the treatment of ALL. 3 marks

e. Name two complications of the condition or its treatment. 2 marks

12) A 6-year-old girl presents to the emergency department with multiple injuries which you cannot explain. She is withdrawn and you are concerned about the nature of the injuries and whether they are related to abuse.

a. Name the four types of abuse. 2 marks

b. Give three risk factors for abuse. 3 marks

c. Name two ways in which maltreatment of a child can come to the 2 marks
   attention of a doctor.

d. Name two specific features in a child with fracture(s) that would make 2 marks
   you suspect abuse.

e. Name one agency that can be accessed in suspected abuse cases. 1 mark

13) A 4-year-old girl presents to the emergency department with a 24-hour history of spiking temperatures, confusion and drowsiness. Her parents have noticed a change in skin colour with mottling of her arms and legs. A rash is present on her feet. You are concerned about meningococcal septicaemia.

a.   Name two causative organisms of meningitis in this age group.   2 marks

b.   Give three other clinical features of meningitis.   3 marks

c.   Describe the characteristic rash in meningococcal disease.   2 marks

d.   What investigation may confirm the causative organism?   1 mark

e.   Give two pharmacological treatments that could be given.   2 marks

Chapter 6

Psychiatry
QUESTIONS

Single best answer questions

1) A 28-year-old male presents to the emergency department with friends reporting out-of-character behaviour. He has a 5-week history of irritability, sexual disinhibition and auditory hallucinations. Which of the following would lead you to diagnose a manic episode?

a. Auditory hallucinations.
b. Increased sexual energy.
c. Irritability.
d. Over-familiarity.

2) Which of the following is not a first-rank symptom of schizophrenia?

a. Delusional perception.
b. Paranoid delusions.
c. Somatic passivity.
d. Thought withdrawal.

3) A 54-year-old male with bipolar affective disorder and chronic kidney disease on bendroflumethiazide and sertraline is commenced on a new medication during a psychiatric inpatient admission. He starts to feel unwell with malaise and anorexia which progresses to dysarthria and a coarse tremor. What is the most likely cause of his current symptoms?

a. Dehydration.
b. Lithium toxicity.
c. Neuroleptic malignant syndrome.
d. Serotonin syndrome.

4) A 17-year-old male presents to his primary care doctor feeling anxious. He particularly struggles with the fear of embarrassing himself and being judged by other people. He has been falling behind at college as he has been unable to deliver presentations in front of classmates. What is the likely diagnosis?

a. Agoraphobia.
b. Generalised anxiety disorder.
c. Panic disorder.
d. Social phobia.

5) A 37-year-old male is commenced onto a monoamine oxidase inhibitor (MAOI) for panic disorder. You counsel him about the side effects; in particular, the risk of a hypertensive crisis. Which of the following in conjunction with a MAOI can lead to a hypertensive crisis?

a. Dopamine.
b. Noradrenaline.
c. Phenylalanine.
d. Tyramine.

6) A 67-year-old male presents to his primary care doctor with a broad-based, slow shuffling gait and 'freezing' episodes. His wife also reports that his memory has been increasingly forgetful and she is struggling to manage him due to this and new episodes of urinary incontinence. What is the most likely diagnosis?

a. Dementia with Lewy bodies.
b. Multiple system atrophy.
c. Normal pressure hydrocephalus.
d. Parkinson's disease.

7) A 27-year-old female presents to her primary care doctor with low mood; she is assessed and diagnosed with mild depression. Which of the following is not recommended by NICE for the initial management of mild depression?

a. Antidepressant medication.
b. Computerised CBT.
c. Individual guided self-help.
d. Structured group physical activity programme.

8) A 19-year-old female is admitted to an inpatient adult psychiatric ward for management of anorexia nervosa. She has had minimal oral intake for the week prior to admission and her BMI is 15.2kg/m^2. Her ECG shows a prolonged PR interval, widespread T wave flattening and prominent U waves. Which electrolyte abnormality is the most likely cause of the ECG changes?

a. Hyperkalaemia.
b. Hypocalcaemia.
c. Hypokalaemia.
d. Hypomagnesaemia.

9) A 29-year-old male presents to his primary care doctor with low mood and apathy. His partner is present and also reports a change in his behaviour with memory loss, unusual movements and disinhibition. His father died aged 54 years from an autosomal dominant disorder. What is the most likely diagnosis?

a.   Frontotemporal dementia.
b.   Haemochromatosis.
c.   Huntington's disease.
d.   Wilson's disease.

10) A 47-year-old female with a background of borderline personality disorder and chronic pain is commenced onto a tricyclic antidepressant (TCA). Which of the following is not an example of a TCA?

a.   Amitriptyline.
b.   Dosulepin.
c.   Duloxetine.
d.   Lofepramine.

11) A 53-year-old male, acting strangely in a park, is found by a member of the public who calls the police. If he is deemed to be suffering from mental illness and in need of immediate care, which part of the Mental Health Act is used to remove him to a place of safety?

a.   Section 2.
b.   Section 5(2).
c.   Section 135.
d.   Section 136.

12) An 8-year-old male attends the Child and Adolescent Mental Health Services with his parents. They are concerned that he is experiencing tics especially outbursts of obscene language which he does not appear able to control. Which symptom is described by the involuntary outbursts of obscene or inappropriate language?

a.   Coprolalia.
b.   Echolalia.
c.   Echopraxia.
d.   Palilalia.

13) A 72-year-old female is admitted as an emergency to the older adults inpatient psychiatry department with severe depression and nihilistic delusions. She is commenced onto medication but quickly deteriorates on the ward. She is now refusing all oral medication and food and water, and the MDT are concerned that there is a risk to her life. What would you do next to treat her mental health?

a.   Admit to general hospital.
b.   Encourage oral intake and medications.
c.   Intramuscular antipsychotic medication.
d.   Refer for emergency electroconvulsive therapy.

14) A 24-year-old female presents to the emergency department with a deliberate overdose of paracetamol. Which of the following binds with NAPBQI to inactivate it preventing hepatic damage?

a.   Cysteine.
b.   Glutathione.
c.   Glucuronide.
d.   Homocysteine.

15) An 84-year-old female is admitted with a urinary tract infection and confusion. She has become increasingly confused and agitated. You suspect delirium. Which of the following is not a cause of acute confused state?

a. Constipation.
b. Electrolyte imbalance.
c. Increasing age.
d. Opiates.

16) A 65-year-old patient with a past medical history of angina and stroke is admitted to hospital with a psychotic episode. Which of the following investigations should be performed in this patient when considering antipsychotic medication?

a. Chest X-ray.
b. CT head.
c. Echocardiogram.
d. Electrocardiogram.

17) A 38-year-old male presents to his primary care doctor complaining of back pain; he states that he is unable to walk due to the pain and is requesting a sick note. Clinical examination is normal and he is subsequently observed returning to his car without obvious difficulties. Which of the following is the most appropriate term to describe this presentation?

a. Conversion disorder.
b. Hypochondriasis.
c. Malingering.
d. Somatisation.

18) A 67-year-old male presents to the memory services with fluctuating cognitive impairment and visual hallucinations. On further questioning, he has been experiencing vivid dreams and at times acting these out for several years. What is the most likely diagnosis?

a.   Alzheimer's disease.
b.   Dementia with Lewy bodies.
c.   Pick's disease.
d.   Vascular dementia.

19) A 57-year-old male with a background of chronic alcohol excess is seen by his primary care doctor with confusion and ataxia. You suspect Wernicke-Korsakoff syndrome. Which vitamin deficiency leads to this disease?

a.   B12.
b.   Folic acid.
c.   Pyridoxine.
d.   Thiamine.

20) A 79-year-old female is diagnosed with Alzheimer's disease. The family and psychiatry team decide it would be appropriate to commence a cognitive enhancer. Which of the following is recommended by NICE as a monotherapy for severe Alzheimer's disease?

a.   Donepezil.
b.   Galantamine.
c.   Memantine.
d.   Rivastigmine.

21) A 27-year-old female presents to her primary care doctor 4 weeks after giving birth to her third child with low mood, anxiety and difficulty sleeping. She is teary throughout the consultation and has a background of a previous moderate depressive episode. What is the most likely diagnosis?

a. Baby blues.
b. Postnatal depression.
c. Postpartum psychosis.
d. Post-traumatic stress disorder.

22) A 37-year-old female complains of low mood, poor appetite and difficulty sleeping; she has noticed that her symptoms worsen during winter and improve significantly over the summer months. What is the most likely diagnosis?

a. Cyclothymia.
b. Depression.
c. Dysthymia.
d. Seasonal affective disorder.

23) An 83-year-old female with a background of Alzheimer's dementia and frequent falls is admitted to hospital with pneumonia. Her family are concerned that she is significantly more disorientated than her baseline and you suspect it is a delirium. She becomes very distressed and aggressive and attempts to assault other patients. De-escalation techniques are unsuccessful and you plan to initiate medication. Which of the following would be most appropriate to manage delirium in the short term?

a. Diazepam.
b. Haloperidol.
c. Lorazepam.
d. Zopiclone.

Extended matching questions

Personality disorders

a.	Paranoid.	e.	Schizoid.
b.	Dissocial.	f.	Emotionally unstable.
c.	Histrionic.	g.	Anankastic.
d.	Avoidant.	h.	Dependent.

Match the characteristics below with the most suitable disorder of adult personality and behaviour.

1) Experiences intense emotions, fears about abandonment and impulsive, self-harming behaviour.

2) Suspiciousness, a tendency to misconstrue actions of others as hostile and lack of trust looking for signs of betrayal.

3) Likes to be the centre of attention, provocative, theatrical expression of emotions, easily influenced and continuously seeks approval.

4) Puts themselves into dangerous and potentially risky situations without considering the consequences, impulsive and a low threshold for aggression and violence.

5) Sets unrealistic high standards, feelings of perfectionism, preoccupation with details and rigidity.

Psychotropic medications

a. SARI.

b. Atypical antipsychotic.

c. Mood stabiliser.

d. SNRI.

e. Typical antipsychotic.

f. SSRI.

g. Tricyclic antidepressant.

h. Benzodiazepine.

Match the medication below to the class that it belongs to.

6) Risperidone.

7) Venlafaxine.

8) Trazadone.

9) Lithium.

10) Lorazepam.

Stress-related and somatoform disorders

a.	Acute stress reaction.	e.	Hypochondriacal disorder.
b.	Dissociative amnesia.	f.	Somatisation disorder.
c.	Adjustment disorder.	g.	Dissociative convulsions.
d.	Dissociative fugue.	h.	Malingering.

Match the clinical history with the most likely disorder.

11) A 34-year-old male recurrently attends the emergency department with the belief that he has cancer. He is not reassured by normal examination findings and test results.

12) A 25-year-old female has been extensively investigated for abdominal pain, pelvic pain and numbness and tingling in her hands. Clinical examination and investigations have found no identifiable physical cause for her symptoms.

13) The fabrication of symptoms for personal gain.

14) A 38-year-old male is brought to the emergency department by the police having been found wandering and unable to recall his name, address or any other details about himself. He is able to recall the names of the police officers after they introduced themselves. Clinical examination, blood results and CT head are normal. Three days later he is suddenly able to remember his personal details and that his wife has left him recently.

15) This disorder may be misdiagnosed as epilepsy.

Dementia

a. Alzheimer's disease.   e. Vascular dementia.
b. Frontotemporal dementia.   f. Creutzfeldt-Jakob disease.
c. Dementia with Lewy bodies.   g. Dementia in Parkinson's.
d. Normal pressure hydrocephalus.   h. Huntington's disease.

Match the description below with the most likely cause of the dementia.

16) Caused by accumulation of prions.

17) The most common cause of dementia.

18) Inherited disorder caused by trinucleotide repeat expansion.

19) Classically presents with a triad of gait disturbance, dementia and urinary incontinence.

20) Associated with a stepwise deterioration.

Therapy

a.	Flooding.	e.	Family therapy.
b.	Cognitive behavioural therapy.	f.	Eye movement desensitisation.
c.	Sensate focus therapy.	g.	Dialectical behavioural therapy.
d.	Systematic desensitisation.	h.	Interpersonal therapy.

Match the text below to the psychotherapy described.

21) This therapy is a modified version of an existing therapy developed to treat borderline personality disorder.

22) A couple's therapy aiming to build trust and intimacy in a relationship by progressing through stages of touching and feedback.

23) This psychotherapy is recommended alongside trauma-focused cognitive behavioural therapy in the management of post-traumatic stress disorder.

24) Patients are directly exposed to their phobic stimuli at its worst in this therapy.

25) Focuses on relationships and how psychological symptoms are a response to difficulties in social interactions with other people.

Eponymous delusions and syndromes

a.   Cotard delusion.   e.   Fregoli syndrome.

b.   Othello syndrome.   f.   Capgras syndrome.

c.   Wernicke's encephalopathy.   g.   De Clerambault's syndrome.

d.   Ekbom's syndrome.   h.   Korsakoff's syndrome.

Match the description below to the eponymous syndrome.

26)   This syndrome is also known as morbid jealousy and is associated with alcoholism.

27)   The patient believes that a person, often of a higher social standing is in love with them.

28)   This syndrome typically presents with formication.

29)   A person holds the belief that a friend, partner or family member has been replaced by an imposter.

30)   The patient has the delusional belief that parts of their body do not exist or are dead or that they are dead or dying.

Addiction

a.	Methadone.	e.	Varenicline.
b.	Disulfiram.	f.	Buprenorphine.
c.	Acamprosate.	g.	Naltrexone.
d.	Bupropion.	h.	Topiramate.

Match the description with the medication used to manage the addiction.

31) Used to maintain abstinence from alcohol and reduces cravings.

32) This medication has opioid agonist and antagonist properties.

33) The mechanism of action is a selective nicotine-receptor partial agonist.

34) Inhibits the enzyme acetaldehyde dehydrogenase.

35) Typically green in colour and used for the treatment of opioid dependency.

Schizophrenia

a. Thought echo.   e. 3rd person hallucinations.
b. Somatic passivity.   f. Thought broadcast.
c. Thought insertion.   g. Command hallucinations.
d. Delusional perception.   h. 2nd person hallucination.

Match the description below with the symptom described.

36) The belief that others can hear an individual's thoughts.

37) The belief or feeling that the individual's thoughts, sensations and actions are under external control.

38) The feeling that the individual's thoughts are not their own and have been placed into their mind.

39) An example of this phenomena would be: a white van driving past is interpreted as meaning that the police are coming to try and harm the individual.

40) Often occurs as a running commentary, for example, "he is walking to the bathroom".

Thought disorder

a.	Tangentiality.	e.	Word salad.
b.	Perseveration.	f.	Circumstantiality.
c.	Clanging.	g.	Pressure of speech.
d.	Neologisms.	h.	Flight of ideas.

Match the description below to the form of thought disorder.

41) New word formations that have no meaning to anyone other than the speaker.

42) Words are related by similar or rhyming sounds rather than their meaning, e.g. rhyming or alliteration.

43) Random words and phrases that are not apparently linked and are unintelligible.

44) Rapid speech which is difficult to interrupt. The patient feels driven to talk and typically presents with hypomania and mania.

45) Repetition of a word or phrase persistently after the subject has been changed.

Short answer questions

1) A 54-year-old male is admitted to inpatient psychiatry with a 3-month history of progressive decline in the community. He reports problems over this time with his neighbours who he states have been trying to kill him; he knows this is the case as he saw a van drive past this morning. He states that neighbours and people walking past can overhear his thoughts and he attempts to prevent this by staying inside his house for the past 2 weeks. On occasions he reports being able to overhear his neighbours commenting on his actions such as "he's now walking to the bathroom". You suspect a relapse of schizophrenia.

a. State three symptoms of schizophrenia that are described above.   3 marks
b. Give two subtypes of schizophrenia.   2 marks
c. Give two examples of typical antipsychotic medications.   2 marks
d. State the four extrapyramidal side effects that are associated with   2 marks
    antipsychotic use.
e. Which atypical antipsychotic has been demonstrated to be efficacious   1 mark
    in treatment-resistant schizophrenia?

2) A 52-year-old male attends his community mental health team for follow-up. He has a background of bipolar affective disorder treated with lithium and olanzapine. He has had previous episodes of mania and severe depression where he has attempted to commit suicide. He has spent a large amount of money on gold coins which he believes will make him a millionaire and that he doesn't have time to eat or drink currently as he has so much work to do. The team are concerned that he is experiencing a relapse in his bipolar disorder.

a. Explain the difference between bipolar I and bipolar II disorder.   1 mark

b. Give one feature you may find in each of the following when   4 marks performing a mental state examination in a patient with a manic episode:
   i. behaviour;
   ii. speech;
   iii. mood;
   iv. thoughts.

c. What medication class is olanzapine?   1 mark

d. State two medications other than lithium used as a mood stabiliser.   2 marks

e. Give two risks that you would be concerned about in this patient   2 marks whilst unwell.

3) A 32-year-old female presents to her primary care doctor with her partner who is concerned that she may be depressed. She reports headaches and menstrual irregularities.

a. State the three core symptoms of major depression.   3 marks

b. Specify four common blood tests you could perform if you suspect an   4 marks organic cause and give your reasoning for these tests.

c. Give an example of a scale used for depression screening.   1 mark

d. Using a rating scale, the primary care doctor classes her depressive 1 mark
episode as moderate and plans to organise CBT and commence a
selective serotonin reuptake inhibitor (SSRI). State an example of an
SSRI.

e. Give one common side effect of SSRI medication that you would warn 1 mark
the patient about.

4) A 33-year-old female presents to her primary care doctor
with a difficulty sleeping 2 weeks after her partner
committed suicide. She is teary throughout the
consultation and reports hearing noises at home which
she interprets as hearing him moving around in the house.

a. The stages of grief model by Kübler-Ross describes five stages of grief; 2 marks
state two of these.

b. Define a hallucination. 2 marks

c. Hearing noises at home interpreted as hearing her partner moving 1 mark
around the house is an example of what?

d. Her partner's death is referred to the coroner due to suicide. State 4 marks
four other deaths that should be referred to the coroner.

e. Eight months following her partner's death she continues to feel 1 mark
hopeless and yearn for him. She is unable to work as she remains
incapacitated by grief. What is this presentation known as?

5) A 23-year-old female attends the emergency department
after taking an intentional overdose of paracetamol. She
reports taking 16 x 500mg paracetamol tablets 8 hours
previously. She feels nauseous but is otherwise well in
herself and is very remorseful about the attempt.

a. State four blood tests to establish if hospital admission is required. 2 marks

b. State the drug used to treat paracetamol overdose. 1 mark

c. Name four things that you would ask about in a suicide assessment. 4 marks

d. Give two sources of support that you would advise the patient to contact if she had thoughts of self-harm or suicide in the future.   2 marks

e. If the mental health team assess a high risk of suicide and the patient is refusing to be admitted, what would you request?   1 mark

6) A 36-year-old male is an inpatient on an adult psychiatric ward with a first presentation of a psychotic episode. He is started on olanzapine; however, due to severe agitation he requires multiple doses of intramuscular haloperidol for rapid tranquillisation during 2 days of admission. The nursing staff report developing confusion and an altered gait. You suspect neuroleptic malignant syndrome (NMS).

a. Give three clinical findings you may find on examination in NMS.   3 marks

b. Give two risk factors for NMS.   2 marks

c. Blockade of which receptor is thought to cause NMS?   2 marks

d. You admit the patient to a medical ward. His conscious level is not impaired and there is currently no evidence of haemodynamic compromise. Give two management points for this patient.   2 marks

e. Which class of medications would be appropriate if he remains severely agitated either in oral or intramuscular form?   1 mark

7) A 79-year-old male with a background of Alzheimer's dementia is admitted from a nursing home to a medical ward with pneumonia. He is disorientated to time and place, and is distressed. He is attempting to leave the ward and nursing staff are concerned he lacks the capacity.

a. Under which part of the Mental Capacity Act could this patient be stopped from leaving the hospital?   1 mark

b. There are five principles of the Mental Capacity Act; state two of these.   2 marks

c. What are four questions that need to be answered to test capacity?   4 marks

d. This patient has no family or close friends to represent him; who 1 mark
    should be involved to support and represent the person?

e. What is an advanced decision?   2 marks

8) A 48-year-old male is a current inpatient on the
    psychiatric intensive care unit with a relapse of
    schizophrenia. He has been increasingly agitated
    throughout the day and the nursing staff are concerned
    that he is demonstrating some aggressive behaviours.

a. Give eight physical or behavioural changes indicating aggression.   4 marks

b. State one medication and route that you would offer.   2 marks

c. Following administration of medication he develops an acute dystonic 1 mark
    reaction. What would you prescribe to treat this?

d. His behaviour settles and you complete a physical examination and   1 mark
    ECG. Upon review of his ECG you note a prolonged QTc at 500ms.
    State one complication that can occur due to a prolonged QT.

e. State two causes of a prolonged QT.   2 marks

9) A 26-year-old female presents to her primary care doctor
    with a feeling of excessive anxiety for several months. She
    hasn't noticed any particular triggers and it is starting to
    affect her ability to go to work. She has read about panic
    attacks and wonders whether she could be experiencing
    these.

a. Give four physical manifestations of a panic attack.   4 marks

b. What is panic disorder?   1 mark

c. State two screening tests that can be used to assess anxiety.   2 marks

d. Specify two non-pharmacological management options for a   2 marks
    generalised anxiety disorder.

e. If non-pharmacological management is unsuccessful and medication   1 mark
    is indicated, NICE recommends either a SSRI or venlafaxine. What
    medication class does venlafaxine belong to?

10) A 48-year-old male is known to the substance misuse services with a background of intravenous drug abuse. He is currently on methadone. He drinks 3L of 8% cider daily and has done this for over 20 years. He has engaged well with the services and is keen to stop alcohol altogether.

a. Calculate his weekly alcohol intake in units. 1 mark
b. What are the four questions in the CAGE questionnaire? 2 marks
c. State four features of alcohol dependence. 4 marks
d. Name one medication that should be prescribed as a reducing regime for withdrawal and one vitamin supplementation. 2 marks
e. Give an example of a medication used to reduce alcohol cravings. 1 mark

11) A 14-year-old female presents to her primary care doctor with her parents who are concerned she has been losing weight. They feel this is due to her belief that she is overweight and she has been restricting her diet. The doctor measures her height as 160cm and her weight as 44kg.

a. Calculate this patient's body mass index (BMI). 2 marks
b. State four findings you may find on physical examination. 4 marks
c. The primary care doctor suspects anorexia nervosa. Give two features of this condition other than weight loss. 2 marks
d. State one psychological treatment for anorexia nervosa. 1 mark
e. She deteriorates in the community and loses further weight; she is admitted to the general hospital for artificial feeding. Three days following commencement of feed she complains of muscle weakness and shortness of breath. What complication is likely to have occurred? 1 mark

12) A 28-year-old female presents to her primary care doctor complaining of decreased libido for the last couple of months. She has a background of depression and asthma and takes fluoxetine and a salbutamol inhaler. The doctor performs blood tests which show a raised prolactin at 720ng/ml.

a. Give six other blood tests to investigate loss of libido.   3 marks
b. State two other symptoms due to hyperprolactinaemia.   2 marks
c. The prolactin is only mildly raised and the primary care doctor feels   2 marks
   that the most likely cause of the increase is her antidepressant
   medication. Give two examples of SSRIs not including fluoxetine.
d. State two causes other than medication of increased prolactin.   2 marks
e. Give one other class of psychotropic drugs other than SSRIs that may   1 mark
   cause hyperprolactinaemia.

13) A male is found acting bizarrely in the street late at night by the police. They are concerned that he may have a mental illness and he is taken to a place of safety under Section 136 of the Mental Health Act (MHA).

a. Give one example of a place of safety.   1 mark
b. What section of the MHA gives nurses holding powers if there is an   1 mark
   immediate need to stop a person from leaving hospital?
c. Following the use of a nurse's holding power, an MHA assessment is   2 marks
   undertaken and he is detained under Section 2:
   i.   what is the purpose of detention under Section 2?
   ii. what is the maximum length of detention under Section 2?
d. State four people that are involved in the multidisciplinary team   4 marks
   whilst he is admitted on the ward.
e. What is a community treatment order?   2 marks

Section 2
Answers

Chapter 7

Dermatology
ANSWERS

1) b.
2) d.
3) b.
4) c.
5) a.
6) c.
7) b.
8) a.
9) d.
10) d.
11) c.
12) b.
13) c.
14) d.
15) a.
16) d.
17) b.
18) a.
19) b.
20) c.

21) c.
22) b.
23) d.

Extended matching question answers

1) b

   Primary biliary cirrhosis is 9 times more common in females and typically presents with fatigue and itching; it may present later with jaundice. Anti-mitochondrial antibodies are found in 90% with primary biliary cirrhosis.

2) c

   An AV fistula suggests that this patient undergoes haemodialysis. The most likely cause of itching mentioned above is therefore uraemia secondary to renal failure.

3) e

   A swelling in the neck may suggest thyroid disease or lymphoma. The heat intolerance makes hyperthyroidism the most likely diagnosis.

4) d

   Altered bowel habit in an elderly adult should prompt you to think about colorectal carcinoma. Shortness of breath is a sign of anaemia.

5) g

   The age demographic and characteristic 'rubbery' feeling on examination suggests Hodgkin's lymphoma.

6) d

   Tender, red, discrete nodules are typical of erythema nodosum which may be seen in streptococcal infection, inflammatory bowel disease and acute sarcoidosis.

7) h

Spider naevi blanch on pressure. They are not always pathological; however, the presence of a large number may be found in liver disease.

8) f

Acanthosis nigricans mainly occurs in skin folds and is described as hyperpigmented, hyperkeratotic skin often described as feeling like velvet. It is associated with diabetes mellitus.

9) b

A rash across the bridge of the nose and cheeks sparing the nasolabial folds are typical of the 'butterfly rash' of systemic lupus erythematosus. It may be seen in mitral stenosis.

10) a

The description is of dermatitis herpetiformis, commonly found in patients with coeliac disease. The papules are classically intensely itchy and improve on undertaking a gluten-free diet. Dapsone is also used.

11) d

Koilonychia may be seen in iron deficiency anaemia and is a spoon shape to the nails.

12) e

Terry's nails are a white ground-glass appearance to the nails.

13) a

Splinter haemorrhages may be found in infective endocarditis; however, they are more commonly due to trauma.

14) g

Linear melanonychia is the descriptive term for subungual melanoma.

15) b

Many nail changes may be present in psoriasis. Out of the options presented above, nail pitting is associated with psoriatic disease.

16) h

Papules can be found in many viral diseases. The central dimple is classical of molluscum contagiosum which usually self-resolves.

17) b

The sandpaper rash and strawberry tongue are characteristics of scarlet fever which is a complication of group A streptococcal infection. Red cheeks with pallor around the mouth, pyrexia and skin peeling are signs of scarlet fever. Desquamation is seen in scalded skin syndrome caused by exotoxins in staphylococcal infection.

18) f

Parvovirus B19 is also known as fifth disease/erythema infectiosum and slapped cheek syndrome due to the erythema on the cheeks and sparing of the nose, eyes and mouth areas. Typically, it presents with a minor febrile illness, it may cause miscarriage or foetal abnormality in pregnant women and can provoke an aplastic crisis in patients with haematological disease.

19) d

Honey-coloured crusting is typical of impetigo. It may be primary or secondary on other dermatological conditions such as atopic eczema.

20) a

Cough, coryza and conjunctivitis are the classical prodrome of measles. Koplik spots are pathognomonic.

21) d

The most suitable answer is a diabetic ulcer, although this is also an example of a neuropathic ulcer. The raised HbA1c makes diabetic ulcer the most appropriate answer.

22) h

Arterial ulcers are found in arteriopaths with comorbidities such as diabetes, hypertension, smoking, ischaemic heart disease and peripheral vascular disease, to name a few. The lack of foot pulses indicates a significant degree of peripheral vascular disease. Arterial ulcers are often painful and described as 'punched-out' lesions. Clinically, the ankle brachial pressure index is a useful investigation to determine arterial disease. This is a contraindication to compression bandaging.

23) b

Pressure ulcers most commonly develop in immobile patients such as during a prolonged hospital length of stay and nursing home residents caused by, as the name suggests, prolonged pressure on the skin. The presence of slough does not indicate a bacterial infection; this would be suggested by a purulent discharge, offensive smell, signs of cellulitis or systemic upset.

24) a

Venous ulcers are typically located below the knee and are largely painless. They are often found in patients with a history of leg swelling and/or varicose veins. Obesity is another risk factor as is hypertension which is commonly found in arterial ulcers; however, the rest of the description does not suit this diagnosis.

25) f

The young age and history of loose stools and mouth ulcers suggest there may be an underlying inflammatory bowel disease; this therefore makes pyoderma gangrenosum the most appropriate answer. This is typically very painful, quick growing and surrounded by a violaceous border. This is not typical of a vasculitic ulcer. In an exam question, you would expect a vasculitic rash to also present with purpura and/or livedo reticularis.

26) d

Mongolian blue spots are birthmarks that are usually present at birth or soon afterwards. They are flat ranging, between blue and grey in colour and are often found on the back and the buttocks. It is important that they are noted at birth as it may be difficult to differentiate a Mongolian blue spot with non-accidental injury.

27) e

A port-wine stain is a red skin discolouration due to a vascular abnormality with the capillaries in the skin. Commonly found on the face, it may be a sign of Sturge-Weber syndrome, a congenital neurological disorder.

28) a

Milia are also known as milk spots. They are keratin-filled small cysts that in the newborn self-resolve within a couple of weeks.

29) c

Erythema toxicum neonatorum is characterised by a red, blotchy rash with pustules. It is common and benign, typically resolving over several weeks.

30) g

Cradle cap is a form of seborrheic dermatitis. It presents with greasy, yellow scales and crusts on the scalp.

31) a

Tinea pedis has various patterns; one of these is athlete's foot, and irritation occurs between the toes.

32) b

Pityriasis versicolor is characterised by patches of scales different in colour to the surrounding skin. A wood lamp can be used to aid the diagnosis and it is caused by a *Malassezia* yeast. Pityriasis rosea is not caused by fungal infection; it typically begins with a herald patch developing into a widespread rash with small pink flaky patches in a 'Christmas-tree' formation.

33) h

Oesophageal candidiasis occurs in immunosuppressed individuals such as patients with HIV and can cause dysphagia. Candida commonly also affects localised areas of skin presenting with redness, itching and discomfort and also the mouth and genital area.

34) g

Tinea infections present with raised scaly, red rings with central sparing. Tinea corporis occurs when this presents on the body/trunk. Tinea capitis refers to the head being affected and tinea unguium is disease of the nail.

35) f

Intertrigo is a rash that occurs in bodily skin folds that can be inflammatory, fungal or bacterial in nature.

36) f

Gottron's sign are red, scaly papules that develop over joints, commonly in the hands. They are found in dermatomyositis.

37) a

Auspitz's sign is typically found in psoriasis; it is the appearance of pinpoint bleeding spots when scales are gently removed.

38) d

Cullen's sign is superficial bruising and oedema found around the umbilicus, first described in relation to ruptured ectopic pregnancy. It is now more commonly associated with acute pancreatitis.

39) c

Russell's sign refers to a callus on the back of the hand or the knuckles relating to repeated episodes of self-induced vomiting.

40) h

Hutchinson's sign can refer to a multitude of different clinical signs. In dermatology, it refers to a pigment band the length of the nail extending to involve the nail fold and suggests subungual melanoma.

41) h

Palmar erythema is redness of the palms due to increased levels of oestrogen; it is also found in liver cirrhosis and alcohol excess.

42) b

Telogen is a phase of the hair cycle during which time hair is shed. Telogen effluvium occurs when there is a significant increase in the hairs shed daily and may be particularly noticeable after washing or brushing hair; it can occur after childbirth or other significant triggering events. It typically self-resolves in several months and requires no intervention; it does not cause scarring.

43) g

Cholestatic pruritus is characterised by intense itching in pregnancy with no cutaneous signs on examination and raised levels of bile acids. Polymorphic eruption of pregnancy presents with an itchy, urticarial rash usually in the third trimester.

44) d

Melasma is characterised by hyperpigmented macules and patches often found on the face, commonly occurring in pregnancy.

45) e

Linea nigra is the descriptive term for a dark, vertical band of hyperpigmented skin down the midline of the abdomen. It typically self-resolves several months after birth.

Short answer question answers

1)

a. Any 3 from: 2 marks

- Family history.
- Stress.
- Smoking.

b. Any 2 from: 2 marks

- Nail pitting.
- Onycholysis.
- Sublingual hyperkeratosis.
- Oil-drop sign.

c. Any 3 from: 3 marks

- Emollients.
- Topical steroids.
- Vitamin D analogues.
- Coal tar.
- Vitamin A analogues.
- Dithranol.

d. Any 2 from: 2 marks

- Guttate.
- Pustular.
- Erythrodermic.
- Flexural.

e. Auspitz's sign.   1 mark

2)

a. Asymmetry.   5 marks

Irregular border.

Colour change.

Diameter greater than 6mm.

Evolving lesion.

b. Any 2 from: 2 marks
  - Increasing age.
  - Previous skin cancer.
  - Multiple naevi.
  - Family history.
  - Parkinson's disease.
  - Skin pigmentation (fair skin, freckled complexion, burns easily).

c. Any 1 from: 1 mark
  - Lentigo maligna.
  - Superficial spreading.
  - Nodular.
  - Acral.
  - Lentiginous.

d. TNM staging.   1 mark
e. Breslow thickness.   1 mark

3)

a. Any 4 from: 4 marks
  - Dolor (pain).
  - Calor (heat).
  - Rubor (redness).
  - Tumour (swelling).
  - Loss of function.

b. Any 2 from: 2 marks
  - *Streptococcus pyogenes.*
  - *Staphylococcus aureus.*
  - Anaerobes.
  - *Pseudomonas aeruginosa.*
  - *Haemophilus influenzae.*
  - *Enterobacteriae.*

c. Necrotising fasciitis.   1 mark
d. Diabetes mellitus.   1 mark

e. Any 4 from: 2 marks
   - Full blood count.
   - Urea & Electrolytes.
   - Glucose/HbA1c.
   - CRP.
   - Blood cultures.
   - Clotting screen.
   - Cross-match.

4)

a. Urticaria.   2 marks
   IgE mediated.

b. Any 3 from: 3 marks
   - Antihistamines.
   - Corticosteroids.
   - Adrenaline.
   - IV fluids.

c. Allergy clinic.   2 marks
   Any 1 from:
   - Skin prick.
   - Fluoroimmunoassay.
   - Radioallergosorbent test (RAST).

d. Any 2 from: 2 marks
   - Avoid known triggers.
   - Advice on EpiPen® use.
   - Always to carry an EpiPen®.
   - Always call an ambulance if symptoms develop.
   - Risk of biphasic reaction.

e. ACE inhibitors, e.g. ramipril.   1 mark

5)

a.   Coeliac disease.   1 mark

b.   Any 1 from: 1 mark

- IgA deposits.
- Subepidermal blisters.
- Inflammatory cells in dermal papillae.

c.   Any 2 from: 2 marks

- Gluten-free diet.
- Dapsone.
- Systemic steroids.

d.   Any 8 from: 4 marks

- FBC.
- U&E.
- LFTs.
- Calcium.
- B12.
- Folate.
- Iron profile.
- Thyroid function.
- Anti-TTG antibodies.
- Anti-endomysial antibodies.
- Gliadin antibodies.
- Immunoglobulins.

e.   Any 2 from: 2 marks

- Alopecia areata.
- Thyroid disease.
- Vitiligo.
- Pernicious anaemia.
- Type 1 diabetes mellitus.
- Addison's disease.

6)

a. Strength (ABV) x Volume (ml)/1000 = 10 units/day, 70 units/week. 1 mark

b. Have you ever felt that you need to cut down on your drinking? 2 marks
    Have you ever felt annoyed by people criticising your drinking?
    Have you ever felt guilty about drinking?
    Have you ever needed a drink first thing in the morning?

c. Any 4 from: 4 marks
    - Facial redness.
    - Flushing.
    - Telangiectasia.
    - Hyperpigmentation.
    - Bruising.
    - Spider naevi.
    - Palmar erythema.
    - Caput medusae.
    - Jaundice.

d. Any 2 from: 2 marks
    - Clubbing.
    - Koilonychia.
    - Terry's nails.
    - Leukonychia.

e. Acetaldehyde. 1 mark

7)

a. Any 3 from: 3 marks
    - Open comedones.
    - Closed comedones.
    - Papules.
    - Pustules.
    - Nodules.
    - Cysts.

b. Any 3 from: 3 marks
    - Topical benzoyl peroxide.
    - Topical antibiotics.

- Topical retinoids.
- Oestrogen contraceptive pill.
- Oral antibiotics.

c. Retinoid.   1 mark

d. Any 2 from: 2 marks
    - Social isolation.
    - Anxiety.
    - Depression.
    - Scarring.
    - Infection.

e. Polycystic ovary syndrome.   1 mark

8)

a. Erythema migrans.   1 mark

b. *Borrelia burgdorferi.*   3 marks
    Spirochete.

c. Any 2 from: 2 marks
    - Facial palsy.
    - Meningitis.
    - Cranial nerve palsy.
    - Encephalitis.
    - Arthritis.
    - Myocarditis.
    - Pericarditis.
    - Uveitis.
    - Hepatitis (there are many other neurological manifestations).

d. Jarisch-Herxheimer reaction.   2 marks

e. Any 2 from: 2 marks
    - Stick to paths.
    - Avoid walking through bushes.
    - Avoid wooded areas.
    - Keep arms and legs covered.
    - Use insect repellent.
    - Monitor skin regularly.

9)

a. Any 3 from: 3 marks
    - Cracked lips.
    - Strawberry tongue.
    - Inflamed buccal mucosa.
    - Desquamation of hands and feet.
    - Erythema/oedema to hands and feet.
    - Rash (may look like measles).

b. Any 3 from: 3 marks
    - Scalded skin syndrome.
    - Measles.
    - Rubella.
    - Scarlet fever.
    - Systemic onset juvenile idiopathic arthritis.
    - Drug reaction, e.g. Stevens-Johnson syndrome.

c. IV immunoglobulin.   1 mark

d. Aspirin.   1 mark

e. There is a risk of coronary artery abnormalities, aneurysms and   2 marks
    stenosis which can lead to cardiac events such as infarction and
    death.

10)

a. Any 4 from: 4 marks
    - Protection.
    - Thermoregulation.
    - Homeostasis.
    - Sensation.
    - Immunological.
    - Vitamin D production.

b. Epidermis.   3 marks
    Dermis.
    Subcutaneous tissue.

c. Collagen and connective tissue production and deposition.   1 mark

d.   Any 1 from: 1 mark

- Eccrine sweat gland.
- Apocrine sweat gland.

e.   Pacinian corpuscle.   1 mark

11)

a.   Anagen.   3 marks
Catagen.
Telogen.

b.   Traction alopecia.   1 mark

c.   Any 2 from: 2 marks

- Psychological distress.
- Social problems.
- Sunburn.
- Permanent hair loss.

d.   Any 3 from: 3 marks

- Alopecia areata.
- Eczema.
- Tinea capitis.
- Lichen planus.
- Psoriasis.
- Seborrheic dermatitis.
- Impetigo.
- Cutaneous lupus erythematosus.
- Cutaneous T-cell lymphoma.

e.   Any 1 from: 1 mark

- Minoxidil.
- Finasteride.

12)

a.   Atopy is the tendency or predisposition to develop allergic or 1 mark
hypersensitive medical conditions.

b. Any 2 from: 2 marks
    ● Hayfever.
    ● Allergic rhinitis.
    ● Asthma.
    ● Food allergies.
    ● Medication allergies.

c. Any 4 from: 4 marks
    ● Irritants, e.g. soap, certain fabrics.
    ● Superimposed infection.
    ● Temperature changes.
    ● Physical contact with allergens.
    ● Inhalation of allergens.
    ● Dietary factors.
    ● Stress.
    ● Hormonal fluctuations.
    ● Dry skin.

d. Any 2 from: 2 marks
    ● Avoid triggers.
    ● Emollients.
    ● Topical steroids.
    ● Antihistamines.

e. Erythroderma.   1 mark

13)

a. Actinic keratosis.   1 mark

b. Biopsy.   1 mark

c. Any 3 from: 3 marks
    ● Cryotherapy.
    ● Excision.
    ● Curettage and electrocautery.
    ● Diclofenac gel.
    ● 5-fluorouracil cream.
    ● Imiquimod cream.

- Photodynamic therapy.
- Ingenol mebutate gel.

d.   Any 3 from: 3 marks

- Occurring in a sun-exposed area.
- Pearly colour.
- Rolled edge.
- Ulcerated centre.
- Telangiectasia.

e.   Any 2 from: 2 marks

- Stay indoors or in the shade in the middle of the day.
- Wear covering clothing.
- High-factor sun cream.
- Avoid sun beds.
- Seek early medical advice if there is concern about a lesion.

Chapter 8

Obstetrics & gynaecology
ANSWERS

Single best answers

1) b.
2) b.
3) d.
4) c.
5) d.
6) a.
7) b.
8) a.
9) b.
10) c.
11) b.
12) b.
13) d.
14) a.
15) c.
16) b.
17) a.
18) a.
19) a.
20) a.

21) d.
22) c.
23) a.

Extended matching question answers

1) d

    Abdominal trauma, especially seatbelt trauma, can cause separation of the placenta from the uterine wall which causes bleeding; this can be apparent (vaginal bleeding) or hidden.

2) g

    Occasionally, women can have endometrial cells present on the cervix often more apparent in pregnancy, which presents as post-coital bleeding and small quantities of vaginal bleeding.

3) e

    The fetal vessels can form over the membranes near the cervical os; when the membranes rupture these vessels also rupture causing massive fetal haemorrhage.

4) h

    The failing pregnancy can bleed into the uterus and cause vaginal bleeding and abdominal pain.

5) a

    Usually placenta praevia is detected earlier in pregnancy and closely monitored. It can cause intermittent bleeding throughout pregnancy and when labour starts this can result in massive haemorrhage.

6) b

    Postpartum infection is a common cause of increased vaginal bleeding and usually results from small amounts of retained products.

7) g

The return of normal menstruation can occur as soon as 4 weeks post-birth; this bleeding can be heavier than previous periods and can be irregular for several months.

8) d

Rectovaginal fistulas are a rare complication of tears and if they are missed they can cause vaginal infections.

9) f

It is normal to pass some blood-stained discharge for a few weeks following childbirth but this usually reduces. It is only a concern if the discharge increases or become foul-smelling.

10) e

Common vaginal infections can occur in postpartum women and should also be considered.

11) a

Incidental cysts that are less than 3mm diameter are physiological cysts and usually resolve spontaneously.

12) e

A type of benign tumour which most commonly occurs in the perimenopausal period and is associated with Meigs syndrome.

13) d

These cysts are usually benign and can contain teratomas which consist of different tissues such as hair, teeth and skin.

14) g

Endometrial tissue in endometriosis can become enclosed in cysts and have a typical ground-glass appearance on ultrasound.

15) b

The pressure of a large fibroid uterus can cause urinary frequency and bloating. The increased endometrial surface area of an enlarged uterus can cause menorrhagia.

16) c

Stressful situations, excessive exercise, significant weight loss and chronic illness can cause hypothalamic failure leading to amenorrhoea. This usually resolves when the causative factor has resolved.

17) d

Hypovolaemia during PPH can cause infarction and pituitary necrosis.

18) g

A LLETZ procedure is where a cone-shaped section of the cervical os is removed; when this heals it can cause the opening to the uterus to become stenosed and the menstrual blood cannot flow out.

19) a

Prolactinomas can cause bitemporal hemianopia, which removes the peripheral vision. Prolactin inhibits the menstrual cycle.

20) e

Thyroid disorders can cause menstrual disorders such as amenorrhoea.

21) g

A sexually transmitted infection that causes painful ulcer-type lesions.

22) e

An autoimmune condition that is most common in postmenopausal women and causes white patches which can be itchy.

23) c

Well-defined vulval lesions are usually associated with cancer elsewhere.

24) a

A pre-cancerous lesion associated with the HPV virus and can be present concurrently with CIN.

25) f

Psoriasis can occur on all areas of skin, and areas that are non-keratinized tend to form smooth lesions.

26) c

Genotypically male but there is insensitivity to the androgens so the Wolffian ducts do not develop and the Mullerian ducts develop.

27) e

XXY; the additional X chromosome causes the secondary sexual characteristics to not develop.

28) g

A condition where there are low levels of sex steroids and gonadotrophins, which causes delayed puberty and poorly developed sexual characteristics.

29) a

A single X chromosome, causes infertility, short stature and a number of congenital malformations.

30) h

The Müllerian duct fails to develop so there is an absent uterus and variable portions of the upper part of the vagina develop.

31) f

These are the most common type of ovarian tumours and serous types are the most common type of epithelial tumour.

32) a

Pseudomyxomas occur when the causative tumour and mucin produced fills the abdominal cavity and can suppress the bowel.

33) h

Benign sex cord stromal tumours that are associated with Meigs syndrome — a triad of tumour, ascites and pleural effusion.

34) b

A tumour that usually forms in the womb and develops from a molar pregnancy but it can also rarely form a solid unilateral ovarian tumour; it is associated with high levels of β-HCG.

35) d

A type of germ cell tumour that is associated with some chromosomal abnormalities which cause abnormal gonads.

36) a

These cells protect the developing spermatozoa prior to being secreted into the seminiferous tubules.

37) f

The primary role of the Leydig cells is to produce androgens.

38) c

The mitotic division of the sperm cells occurs under the influence of FSH in the Sertoli cells.

39) b

The final stage of sperm cell maturation occurs under LH influence.

40) h

These are the first gonadotrophs in the production of sperm.

41) f

This is an abnormality where the bowel fails to return to the body following its development. This condition has a better prognosis as it is usually an isolated abnormality.

42) b

A condition where there is a narrowing in the aorta and depending on the location of the narrowing there may be a lower blood pressure observed in the lower limbs in comparison with the upper limbs.

43) g

A small neural tube defect through which the meninges and spinal cord do not perforate the skin. This is often never diagnosed but can be seen as a small hairy patch or a dimple in the skin.

44) h

The ductus arteriosus should close at birth; when this is patent it allows oxygenated blood in the arterial system to pass into the pulmonary circulation causing a peripheral cyanosis.

45) a

A condition which is classified as the presence of four different cardiac abnormalities: overriding aorta, pulmonary stenosis, right ventricular hypertrophy and ventricular septal defect. When the baby increases its oxygen demand by crying it becomes hypoxic.

Short answer question answers

a. Any 4 from: 4 marks
    - Orofacial defects.
    - Neural tube defects.
    - Congenital heart defects.
    - Haemorrhagic disease of the newborn.

b. Status epilepticus.   2 marks
    Sudden unexpected death in epilepsy.

c. Folic acid 5mg.   2 marks

d. Increased hepatic metabolism and increased renal clearance causes   1 mark
    decreased levels of antiepileptic drugs.

e. Breastfeeding is not affected and so is encouraged.   1 mark

2)

a. Heavy cyclical periods which interfere with physical, social or   1 mark
    emotional quality of life or menstrual bleeding >80ml.

b. Any 1 from: 2 marks
    - Systemic: thyroid disease, clotting disorders.

    Any 1 from:
    - Local: fibroids, polyps, endometrial carcinoma, endometriosis,
      pelvic inflammatory disease, dysfunctional uterine bleeding.

c. Any 1 from: 1 mark
    - Fatigue.
    - Breathlessness.
    - Chest pain.

d. Any 1 from: 2 marks
    - Serum: FBC, TFTs, clotting.

    Any 1 from:
    - Physical: ultrasound, endometrial biopsy, hysteroscopy.

e. Any 2 from: 4 marks
    ● With contraception: oral progestogens, Mirena coil (IUS),
      combined oral contraceptive pill, danazol, GnRH agonists.
    Any 2 from:
    ● Without contraception: tranexamic acid, aspirin, indomethacin,
      mefenamic acid.

3)

a. Endometrial tissue that is present outside of the uterine cavity.   1 mark

b. During menstruation endometrial tissue is spilt into the pelvic cavity   2 marks
    via the Fallopian tubes (retrograde menstruation) (1 mark); this
    implants and becomes functional responding to ovarian cycle
    hormones (1 mark).

c. Any 2 from: 2 marks
    ● Ovaries.
    ● Pouch of Douglas.
    ● Uterosacral ligaments.

d. Diagnostic laparoscopy.   1 mark

e. Any 4 from: 4 marks
    ● Combined contraceptive pill.
    ● Progestogens.
    ● Mirena coil.
    ● GnRH agonists.
    ● Gestrinone.
    ● Danazol.
    ● Surgical management.

4)

a. β-HCG.   3 marks
    CA125.
    AFP.

b. Any 1 from: 1 mark
    ● BRCA1.
    ● BRCA2.

c. Any 2 from: 2 marks
    - HRT.
    - Nulliparous.
    - White Caucasian.
    - Blood group A.
    - Late age of first conception.
    - Family history.
    - Increasing age.
    - Obesity.
    - Early menarche.
    - Late menopause.
    - Smoking.
d. Epithelial.   3 marks
    Sex cord stromal.
    Germ cell.
e. Any 1 from: 1 mark
    - Liver.
    - Lung.

5)

a. Stress incontinence.   1 mark
b. Any 3 from: 3 marks
    - Puborectalis.
    - Pubococcygeus.
    - Iliococcygeus.
    - Coccygeus.
    - Levator ani.
    - Piriformis.
    - Sacrospinatous.
c. Any 2 from: 2 marks
    - Multiparity.
    - Raised intra-abdominal pressure.
    - Menopause.

- Hysterectomy.
- Prolonged second stage of labour.

d. Any 2 from: 2 marks
- Avoiding prolonged second stage of labour.
- Appropriate use of instrumental deliveries and episiotomy.
- Pelvic floor exercises.
- Support of vaginal vault during hysterectomy.

e. Any 1 from: 2 marks
- Conservative: use of pessaries, physiotherapy.

Any 1 from:
- Surgical: anterior repair for cystocele, posterior repair for rectocele.

6)

a. Acute: premature rupture of membranes.   2 marks

Any 1 from:
- Chronic: renal agenesis, fetal abnormality, aneuploidy, IUGR, fetal infection, amnion nodosum.

b. Any 2 from: 2 marks
- Pulmonary hypoplasia.
- Respiratory difficulties.
- Club foot.
- Skull deformities.
- Wry neck.
- IUGR.

c. Any 2 from: 2 marks
- Umbilical cord compression.
- Fetal hypoxia.
- Shoulder dystocia.

d. Deepest pool of amniotic fluid <2cm.   2 marks
Ultrasound.

e. Encouraging maternal hydration.   2 marks
Amnioinfusion.

7)

a. Any 3 from: 3 marks
- Oedema.
- Swelling.
- Visual disturbance.
- Right upper quadrant pain.
- Epigastric pain.

b. Any 2 from: 2 marks
- Urine dipstick for protein.
- Urine protein: creatinine ratio.
- LFTs.
- Full blood count.
- Clotting.
- U&Es.

c. New hypertension occurring after 20 weeks' gestation with significant proteinuria. 1 mark

d. HELLP syndrome. 1 mark

e. Haemolysis. 3 marks
Elevated LFTs.
Low platelets.

8)

a. 1st stage — from onset of labour to full cervical dilatation. 3 marks
2nd stage — from full cervical dilatation to expulsion of the fetus.
3rd stage — from fetus expulsion to delivery of the placenta.

b. 1cm per hour. 1 mark

c. Any 3 from: 3 marks
- Transcutaneous electrical nerve stimulation (TENS).
- Acupuncture.
- Massage.
- Hypnosis.
- Relaxation techniques.
- Diamorphine.

- Pethidine.
- Entonox.
- Epidural.

d. Ischial spines. 1 mark

e. Physiological — the cord is not cut until it ceases to pulsate and the placenta is delivered passively. 2 marks

Active — the cord is clamped and cut, an oxytocic drug is used and controlled cord traction is used to remove the placenta.

9)

a. Nuchal translucency. 4 marks

AFP.

β-HCG.

Unconjugated estriol.

b. Down's syndrome — trisomy 21. 3 marks

Edwards syndrome — trisomy 18.

Patau's syndrome — trisomy 13.

c. Any 1 from: 1 mark

- Amniocentesis (15-20 weeks).
- Chorionic villous sampling (11-14 weeks).

d. Surgical evacuation of the uterus. 1 mark

e. Rhesus status — if Rhesus negative, the patient will require anti-D. 1 mark

10)

a. Failure to conceive after 2 years of regular unprotected intercourse. 1 mark

b. Any 2 from: 2 marks

- Cystic fibrosis.
- Epididymo-orchitis.
- History of STI.
- Post-pubertal mumps.

c. Any 1 from: 3 marks
- Ovulatory: chronic systemic illness, eating disorder, PCOS, hyperprolactinaemia, thyroid disease.

Any 1 from:
- Tubal: PID, tubal surgery, previous ectopic, endometriosis.

Any 1 from:
- Uterine: fibroids, septae, congenital, Asherman syndrome.

d. Ultrasound pelvis.   2 marks

Hysterosalpingogram.

e. Any 2 from: 2 marks
- Motility.
- Progression.
- Morphology.
- Number.
- Volume.

11)

a. Antihistamine, e.g. cyclizine.   1 mark

b. Complete mole (1 mark) — caused by the combination of an anuclear   4 marks egg and either one or two sperm (if one, this then duplicates), producing a trophoblast containing only paternal DNA which is always diploid (1 mark).

Incomplete mole (1 mark) — caused by the combination of a haploid egg with either two sperm or one sperm which subsequently duplicates causing a triploid or tetraploid trophoblast (1 mark).

c. β-HCG.   1 mark

d. Chorioadenoma — benign.   2 marks

Choriocarcinoma — malignant.

e. Surgical curettage (1 mark) and follow-up with regular β-HCG every 2   2 marks weeks for the first 8 weeks, then every 3 months for 6 months to 2 years (1 mark).

12)

a. Vaginal cephalic delivery (1 mark) which requires additional obstetric   3 marks
manoeuvres to deliver the body once the head is delivered (1 mark),
due to the anterior shoulder becoming impacted on the symphysis
pubis (1 mark).

b. Any 1 from: 3 marks
    - Maternal: diabetes, high BMI, short stature, previous history.
    Any 1 from:
    - Fetal: estimated fetal weight >4500g, >42 weeks' gestation.
    Any 1 from:
    - Interventional: induction or augmentation of labour.

c. McRoberts manoeuvre.   2 marks
    Suprapubic pressure.

d. Any 1 from: 1 mark
    - Brachial plexus injury.
    - Hypoxic brain injury.
    - Fetal death.

e. Any 1 from: 1 mark
    - Postpartum haemorrhage.
    - 3rd/4th degree tears.
    - Uterine rupture.

13)

a. 1-3 weeks.   1 mark

b. Any 3 from: 3 marks
    - Atypical skin scarring.
    - IUGR.
    - Cataracts.
    - Cerebral cortical atrophy.
    - Global developmental delay.

c. Respiratory droplets.   2 marks
    Contact with vesicular fluid either directly or indirectly.

d. Live attenuated virus. 2 marks
No, this can cause fetal infection.

e. Varicella zoster immunoglobulin. 2 marks
IM injection.

Chapter 9

Oncology
ANSWERS

Single best answers

1) c.
2) a.
3) b.
4) d.
5) b.
6) b.
7) d.
8) a.
9) c.
10) d.
11) d.
12) a.
13) a.
14) a.
15) b.
16) d.
17) d.
18) b.
19) b.
20) d.

21) a.
22) a.
23) d .

Extended matching question answers

1) b

CA-125 is used as a tumour marker for ovarian cancer. It is also used for risk stratification of ovarian cysts.

2) f

CEA is the tumour marker used to monitor and check for recurrence of colorectal cancer. CEA is a glycoprotein from gastrointestinal epithelia.

3) h

β-HCG can be used to monitor the response of choriocarcinoma to treatment, or to monitor untreated disease. β-HCG is disproportionately high in patients with choriocarcinoma as it consists of syncytiotrophoblasts (these produce β-HCG).

4) a

Alpha-fetoprotein is characteristically raised in patients with non-seminomatous germ cell tumours.

5) e

Medullary cell carcinoma of the thyroid is a neuroendocrine tumour of calcitonin producing C-cells; therefore, calcitonin levels are found to be high.

6) e

A complete response means disappearance of all radiological signs of cancer in response to treatment; this is not equivocal to cure.

7) d

Cancer that is spreading or growing is defined as progressive disease.

8) b

Disease-free survival means the length of time following treatment without symptoms or signs of disease.

9) a

Following completion of treatment, the disease remaining is described as residual disease.

10) c

After 5 years the percentage of patients alive can be described as overall survival.

11) a

Cushing's syndrome is a well-described phenomenon in small cell lung cancers; it is caused by ectopic ACTH production.

12) e

Carcinoid syndrome can be caused by neuroendocrine tumours. Typical symptoms include: flushing, diarrhoea, breathlessness, cramps and nausea/vomiting.

13) a

SIADH is commonly associated with small cell lung cancer. Hyponatraemia can cause drowsiness, confusion and seizures.

14) c

Phaeochromocytomas are tumours of the sympathetic nervous system. Headache, sweating and palpitations are seen in over 90% of cases. Symptoms are produced by hormones produced by the tumours.

15) g

Germ cell tumours are often found to cause gynaecomastia.

16) a

Stereotactic radiosurgery can be used to treat small tumours; it delivers targeted radiation at high doses to a specific area of the brain. It is used to maintain function and usually for palliation.

17) c

White out lung in this context has two differentials: lung collapse, and consolidation or significant pleural effusion. If the lung was collapsed the trachea would be deviated towards the affected lung. The trachea is deviated away, so this is consistent with pleural effusion. Symptomatic pleural effusion should be managed with a chest drain.

18) e

The history of pyrexia and features of sepsis following chemotherapy should indicate possible neutropenic sepsis.

19) f

Liver capsule pain is often described by patients with liver metastases. Treatment by steroids reduces the volume of liver metastases. Other analgesia may still be indicated.

20) d

The history is suspicious for hypercalcaemia; this electrolyte imbalance is often seen in prostate cancer. The main treatment for hypercalcaemia is aggressive fluid resuscitation, and bisphosphonates can be given intravenously every 7 days.

21) b

Treatment given after the primary treatment is called adjuvant treatment. This is used to reduce the risk of recurrence.

22) e

When a sealed radioactive source is placed into a bodily cavity, this is known as radiation brachytherapy.

23) a

Treatment aiming for cure is called radical treatment.

24) h

Phase 3 clinical trials compare the efficacy of a drug versus the current available treatments. Phase 1 and 2 trials are designed to test for drug safety.

25) f

Phase 1 trials assess the safety of new drugs in humans.

26) a

Pyrexia within 6 weeks of chemotherapy should make you suspicious of neutropenic sepsis. This should be treated aggressively as it has a high mortality rate.

27) f

Coronary spasm is a known side effect of 5-fluorouracil and capecitabine chemotherapy; it can cause arrhythmias and myocardial infarction. If this occurs, the patient should be managed as any other cardiac chest pain and the infusion should be stopped.

28) b

Extravasation describes leakage of fluid into the surrounding tissues. Injuries can be caused by irritant drugs; if chemotherapy agents are particularly vesicant they can cause significant tissue injury requiring plastic surgeon involvement.

29) h

Renal cell carcinoma frequently causes anaemia. This patient has symptoms of anaemia likely requiring a blood transfusion.

30) e

Chemotherapy given for large bulk chemosensitive tumours can often cause tumour lysis syndrome. Patients often develop severe electrolyte disturbances and renal failure. Allopurinol and rasburicase can be used as prophylaxis to prevent tumour lysis syndrome.

31) g

Multiparity is protective against ovarian cancer.

32) a

Schistosomiasis is associated with squamous cell bladder cancer. The most common histology of bladder cancer is transitional cell carcinoma.

33) e

Barrett's oesophagus is a dysplastic condition in which gastric mucosa develops in the oesophagus. Patients with this are prone to developing oesophageal carcinoma and require regular screening.

34) d

H. pylori infection predisposes to the development of gastric cancer. It is treated with proton pump inhibitors (PPIs) and antibiotics.

35) f

Late menopause is associated with endometrial cancer as the uterus is exposed to oestrogen for an increased number of years.

36) e

Between the ages of 25 and 49 women should be screened every 3 years; if patients are high risk they are screened more frequently.

37) e

Between the ages of 50 and 70 years, women should have mammograms every 3 years.

38) b

Between ages 50 and 64 years, women should have cervical screening every 5 years.

39) g

High-grade CIN (cervical intraepithelial neoplasia) is best investigated using colposcopy. This is more sensitive and can be used to determine if any treatment is indicated.

40) c

People between the age of 60 and 74 should be screened regularly for bowel cancer using the faecal occult blood test. This looks for the presence of blood in multiple stool samples. Patients with a positive result may be invited for colonoscopy. If the result is unclear, patients are asked to repeat the test.

41) h

There are several types of multiple endocrine neoplasia. MEN-1 is associated with parathyroid tumours, pituitary adenomas and pancreatic tumours.

42) d

Von Hippel-Lindau syndrome is associated with retinal angioma, phaeochromocytoma, renal cell carcinoma and cerebellar/spinal haemangiomas.

43) e

Familial adenomatous polyposis is a condition associated with a mutation in the APC tumour suppressor gene. Patients develop multiple bowel adenomas and frequently develop colorectal cancer at an early age. These patients require frequent screening.

44) f

Li-Fraumeni syndrome is an autosomal dominant condition resulting in the inactivation of the P53 gene which usually acts to downregulate the cell cycle to regulate apoptosis. These patients often develop breast carcinoma, sarcoma and some brain tumours.

45) e

Patients with Peutz-Jeghers syndrome develop multiple hamartomatous polyps in the gastrointestinal tract. They often have mucocutaneous pigmentation. The polyps are prone to malignant transformation.

Short answer question answers

1)

a. Two or more criteria of a systemic inflammatory response syndrome   2 marks
    (SIRS) (1 mark) with a documented source of infection (1 mark).

b. Fluids.   3 marks
    Antibiotics.
    Blood cultures.
    Catheter.
    Lactate.
    Oxygen.

c. Any 4 from: 2 marks
    - Chest X-ray.
    - Urine dip.
    - Mid-stream urine.
    - Hickman line cultures.
    - Peripheral blood cultures.

d. Broad-spectrum antibiotics, e.g. Tazocin + gentamycin.   1 mark

e. Line removal.   2 marks

2)

a. Any 2 from: 2 marks
    - *C. difficile*.
    - Rotavirus.
    - Adenovirus.
    - Norovirus.

b. CT abdomen.   1 mark
    Abdominal X-ray.

c. Immune-mediated colitis secondary to pembrolizumab.   2 marks

d. Hypomagnesaemia.   3 marks
    Hypokalaemia.
    Hyponatraemia.

e. Any 2 from: 2 marks
    - IV steroids.
    - IV fluids.
    - Electrolyte replacement.

3)
a. Transitional cell carcinoma.   2 marks
b. Any 3 from: 3 marks
    - Schistosomiasis.
    - Azo dye.
    - Rubber manufacturing.
    - Smoking.
c. Cystectomy and reconstruction/urostomy formation.   1 mark
d. Any 2 from: 2 marks
    - IV fluids.
    - Stopping nephrotoxic drugs.
    - Monitor urine output.
e. Left-sided nephrostomy.   2 marks
    Left ureteric stent insertion.

4)
a. Any 3 from: 3 marks
    - Previous head and neck radiation.
    - Alcohol.
    - HPV.
    - Smoking.
    - Chewing tobacco/betel nuts.
b. Squamous cell carcinoma.   1 mark
c. Treatment with curative intent.   3 marks
    Chemoradiotherapy.
d. Mucositis.   1 mark
e. Any 2 from: 2 marks
    - Mouthwashes.
    - Artificial saliva.

- Dietetic input/assessment.
- Nutritional supplementation.
- Analgesia.

5)

a. Any 4 from: 2 marks
- Weight loss.
- Fever.
- Night sweats.
- Saddle paraesthesia.
- Weakness.
- Numbness.
- Faecal incontinence.
- History of malignancy.
- Immunosuppression.

b. Spinal cord compression.   2 marks

c. Any 2 from: 2 marks
- MRI spine.
- Steroids.
- Consideration of surgical stabilisation.

d. Biochemically: prostate-specific antigen.   2 marks
Histological: Gleason score.

e. Surgical castration or chemical castration with a GnRH antagonist   2 marks
such as degarelix.

6)

a. Small cell.   2 marks
Non-small cell (squamous cell, adenocarcinoma, large cell).

b. WHO/Eastern Cooperative Oncology Group Performance Status.   1 mark

c. Grade 2 (1 mark) — restricted in strenuous activity but ambulatory   2 marks
and able to carry out light work, active but with the aid of analgesics
(1 mark).

d. Any 3 from: 3 marks
- Domperidone/metoclopramide — dopamine antagonist.
- Ondansetron/granisetron — 5HT3 (serotonin) antagonist.
- Haloperidol — antipsychotic.
- Cyclizine — antihistamine.

e. Any 2 from: 2 marks
- Persistent vomiting.
- Hypovolaemia.
- SIADH.

7)

a. Bowel cancer. 1 mark
Breast cancer.

b. Any 3 from: 3 marks
- Agreed population.
- Acceptable test.
- Important condition.
- Latent period of disease allows for intervention.
- Natural history is well understood.
- Diagnostic facilities available.
- Appropriate test is available.
- Effective early treatment available.
- Cost-effective.
- Screening needs to be continuous.

c. Specificity — ability to detect negatives. 4 marks
Sensitivity — ability to detect positives.
Lead time bias — overestimation of survival duration due to earlier detection by screening.
Length time bias — overestimation of survival duration due to the relative excess of cases detected that are slowly progressing.

d. HPV 16/18. 1 mark

e. FIGO. 1 mark

8)

a. Any 3 from: 3 marks
- Difficulty breathing.
- Dyspnoea.
- Swollen face.
- Swollen arms.

b. Any 2 from: 2 marks
- Stridor.
- Prominent veins on the chest wall.
- Oedema in the neck and arms.
- Engorged face.

c. CT chest.   1 mark

d. Steroids.   2 marks

e. Radiotherapy.   2 marks
   Stenting procedure.

9)

a. Any 4 from: 2 marks
- Unilateral breast lump.
- Skin tethering.
- Ulceration.
- Nipple discharge.
- Skin discoloration (peau d'orange).
- Weight loss.

b. Palpation.   3 marks
   Fine needle biopsy.
   Imaging (USS).

c. TNM staging.   1 mark

d. Any 4 from: 2 marks
- Malaise.
- Polyuria.
- Nocturia.
- Drowsiness.

- Bone pain.
- Abdominal pain.
- Confusion.
- Dehydration.
- Depression.

e.   IV fluids.   2 marks
     Bisphosphonates.

10)

a.   Any 2 from: 2 marks
   - External beam radiotherapy.
   - Radionucleotides (iodine-131).
   - Brachytherapy.

b.   Fraction — the full dose of radiation is usually divided into a number   1 mark
     of smaller doses called fractions.

c.   Any 4 from: 4 marks
   - Anorexia.
   - Nausea.
   - Malaise.
   - Mucositis.
   - Oesophagitis.
   - Diarrhoea.
   - Alopecia.
   - Sore skin/rash.

d.   Any 2 from: 1 mark
   - Radiotherapy tattoo.
   - Plastic mask.
   - Plastic suit.

e.   Any 2 from: 2 marks
   - Pain management (e.g. bone metastases).
   - Reduction of headache/vomiting with brain metastases.
   - Relief of obstruction (bronchus, superior vena cava, oesophagus).
   - Maintaining skeletal integrity with bone metastases.
   - Management of spinal cord compression.

11)

a. Ovarian cancer causes a few specific symptoms such as vague abdominal discomfort and bloating.   2 marks

b. CA125.   1 mark

c. Simple analgesia — paracetamol/NSAID.   3 marks
Weak opioid — codeine/tramadol.
Strong opioid — morphine/oxycodone.

d. Paracentesis or ascitic drain insertion.   2 marks

e. Any 4 from: 2 marks
- Morphine/oxycodone — pain.
- Haloperidol — nausea.
- Midazolam — agitation.
- Hyoscine butylbromide — secretions.
- Hyoscine hydrobromide — secretions.

12)

a. Bowen's disease.   2 marks
Actinic keratoses.

b. ABCDE criteria.   3 marks
Asymmetrical.
Border irregularity.
Colour variation.
Diameter >6mm.
Elevation.

c. Any 3 from: 3 marks
- Pale skin.
- Multiple melanocytic naevi.
- Family history.
- Sun exposure.
- Immunosuppression.
- Lentigo maligna.
- Giant congenital melanocytic naevi.
- Atypical mole syndrome.

d.   Wide excision.   1 mark

e.   Immunotherapy.   1 mark

13)

a.   Any 2 from: 2 marks

   ● Non-specific symptoms/no symptoms so detected late.

   ● Complete resection is often difficult and rarely curative.

   ● Adjuvant chemotherapy is rarely curative.

b.   In the presence of a palpably enlarged gallbladder (0.5 marks), which   2 marks
      is non-tender (0.5 marks), accompanied with painless jaundice (0.5
      marks), the cause is unlikely to be gallstones (0.5 marks).

c.   TNM system.   1 mark

d.   Epigastric or left upper quadrant.   3 marks

      Radiating to back.

      Improved on leaning forward.

e.   Any 2 from: 2 marks

   ● Ascites.

   ● Superficial migratory thrombophlebitis.

   ● Jaundice.

   ● Pallor.

   ● Hepatomegaly.

   ● Palpable mass in the epigastrium.

Chapter 10

Ophthalmology
ANSWERS

Single best answers

1) a.
2) d.
3) b.
4) b.
5) d.
6) a.
7) c.
8) b.
9) b.
10) c.
11) b.
12) a.
13) d.
14) c.
15) b.
16) d.
17) a.
18) c.
19) a.
20) b.

21)   c.
22)   d.
23)   b.

Extended matching question answers

1) d

A third nerve palsy causes a dilated pupil that fails to react to light or accommodation. Other features such as ptosis and a divergent squint should also be present.

2) e

An Adie's pupil is caused by damage to postganglionic parasympathetic fibres within the orbit, leading to a pupil that reacts slowly to direct light and accommodation, and is slow to redilate.

3) g

Horner's syndrome is caused by damage to sympathetic nerve fibres. If the lesion occurs below the superior cervical ganglion, decreased facial sweating is present; this type of pupil can be differentiated from a normal pupil as 4% cocaine causes dilation of a normal pupil but not a Horner's pupil which will dilate with the administration of 0.1% adrenaline.

4) f

A relative afferent pupillary defect results from damage to the afferent pathway on one side and is detected by the swinging torch test. In a normal test, moving the torch between each eye and back should result in equally constricted pupils due to the direct and consensual light reflexes; however, damage to the afferent pathway will lead to a reduction in constriction on the affected side during the second attempt at a direct consensual reflex compared with the indirect reflex.

5)   b

An Argyll-Robertson pupil is most commonly associated with neurosyphilis but is also present in trauma, tumours or vascular events. Small, unequal irregular pupils will be seen which do not respond to the light reflex but accommodate promptly.

6)   d

Cromoglicate can be used in the treatment of allergic conjunctivitis by stabilising mast cells which act as an anti-inflammatory agent to reduce ocular irritation.

7)   g

Phenylephrine is a selective α-1 adrenergic receptor agonist which stimulates pupillary dilatation in order to allow retinal visualisation.

8)   b

Prostaglandin analogues such as latanoprost act to increase aqueous outflow by the uveoscleral route. Carbonic anhydrase inhibitors such as acetazolamide reduce aqueous secretion by the ciliary body.

9)   f

Fluorescein is used to help identify corneal ulcers as the exposed corneal stroma are stained by this dye making them appear green allowing for identification of the ulcer margins. Dendritic ulcers are associated with the *Herpes simplex* virus.

10) e

Hypromellose is a modified cellulose polymer that is water-soluble and when placed on the ocular surface acts to absorb water, increasing the thickness of the tear film.

11) a

Basal cell carcinomas are the most common tumour encountered in ophthalmology. They most commonly occur on the lower eyelid and have a characteristic pearly appearance with overlying telangiectasia which may bleed or ulcerate. Excision is the treatment of choice.

12) f

A chalazion (meibomian cyst) is a swelling due to a blocked meibomian duct leading to inflammation. Treatment is initially with a warm compress; however, if it is large or it recurs frequently, an incision and curettage may be used. It is important to note that a recurrent chalazion may be a sebaceous gland carcinoma which is highly malignant and in this case an incisional biopsy is required.

13) e

Orbital apex syndrome is the series of cranial nerve dysfunctions due to a lesion at the superior orbital fissure and optic canal. It involves the optic, oculomotor, trochlear abducens and ophthalmic branch of the trigeminal nerve leading to ophthalmalgia, vision loss and ptosis.

14) d

Orbital cellulitis is a life-threatening condition that if not treated promptly can lead to loss of vision. It is usually caused by infection in the paranasal sinuses by organisms such as *Haemophilus influenzae*, *Streptococcus pneumoniae* or anaerobes. It is more common in children and a classic triad of an unwell child with painful restricted eye movements and sinus tenderness will point towards a diagnosis of orbital cellulitis and must be treated with IV antibiotics.

15) b

Melanoma is a malignant tumour of melanocytes and although ocular cancers are rare, melanomas are the most common type. Although the main risk factors for skin melanoma is exposure to UV light, the link between UV and ocular melanoma is unclear. Breslow thickness is a prognostic indicator and is used to determine the surgical margin during excision of the lesion.

16) c

Macular sparing is evident due to collateral circulation from the middle cerebral artery to the macula. The remainder of the visual cortex is supplied by the posterior cerebral artery.

17) b

A lesion of the parietal lobe causes a homonymous inferior quadrantanopia, whereas occipital lesions cause a homonymous superior quadrantanopia.

18) h

A lesion of the right optic tract will lead to a left homonymous hemianopia whereas a lesion to the optic radiation will lead to a quadrantanopia.

19) d

Lesions that affect the eye and optic nerves before the optic chiasm cause visual defects on the same side as the lesion.

20) f

A bitemporal hemianopia is caused by pressure on the optic chiasm disrupting nasal fibres of both optic nerves.

21) b

Ocular tuberculosis is more prevalent in the developing world and is due to infection by *Mycobacterium tuberculosis*. Ocular TB is presumed if findings such as anterior uveitis, granulomatous, mutton-fat keratic precipitates or choroidal tubercles are seen with systemic findings consistent with TB. Ocular TB is treated as pulmonary TB with rifampicin, isoniazid, ethambutol and pyrazinamide for 2 months, then rifampicin and isoniazid for 4 months.

22) d

The patient has an Argyll-Robertson pupil and in conjunction with his neurological symptoms a diagnosis of tertiary syphilis can be made.

23) g

Congenital rubella syndrome is a classic triad of sensorineural deafness, eye pathology and cardiac disease. It is caused by rubella infection during the first 26 weeks of conception.

24) e

Herpes zoster ophthalmicus is caused by the varicella zoster virus and presents as a unilateral painful dermatomal skin rash with pain or numbness around the eye and forehead. It is treated with oral acyclovir.

25) c

Toxocariasis is caused by a roundworm *Toxocara canis* or *Toxocara cati* found in the intestine of dogs or cats. It commonly affects young children as they often come into contact with contaminated material whilst playing outside. Topical steroids and anti-helminth therapies such as albendazole are used to treat this condition.

26) b

The case history describes allergic conjunctivitis. As the patient experienced the same symptoms 12 months ago it can be assumed it is a seasonal type known as vernal keratoconjunctivitis. The cobblestone appearance on the superior tarsal conjunctiva is typical of this variant.

27) e

The history of sudden onset lacrimation whilst at work in a manual labour environment should point towards the possibility of a corneal foreign body. This diagnosis can be reinforced by the patient struggling to open his eye due to pain.

28) g

Endophthalmitis is a rare but serious complication following cataract surgery and is a painful red eye usually with a purulent discharge. Examination may reveal a relative afferent pupillary defect and a hypopyon may be seen. It requires urgent admission for antibiotics.

29) c

The severe pain, presence of vomiting and fixed mid-dilated pupil are all classical signs of acute closed angle glaucoma. Urgent treatment is needed to reduce ocular pressure as permanent visual loss can occur and after the initial event, further treatment such as laser iridotomy on both eyes may be performed to prevent further episodes.

30) h

Scleritis is often associated with systemic disease and is a red and severely painful eye involving all layers of the sclera. This is in comparison to episcleritis with is usually painless and not associated with systemic disease.

31) g

Wilsons's disease is an autosomal recessive disorder due to a mutation in the ATP7B gene resulting in copper accumulation within the body. It can affect many organ systems including the liver, kidneys, brain, heart and eyes. Kayser-Fleischer rings are brownish-yellow rings visible around the limbus and are due to copper deposition within Descemet's membrane within the cornea. Serum ceruloplasmin is low and urinary copper is high. Wilson's disease is treated with penicillamine to chelate copper.

32) d

Multiple sclerosis is a demyelinating disorder of the central nervous system. One third of patients will present with optic neuritis, which is an inflammation of the optic nerve; characteristic findings on fundoscopy are a swollen and pale optic disc. Lhermitte's sign is the electric shock sensation running down the back on bending the neck and is a classical finding in multiple sclerosis.

33) b

Neurofibromatosis is a genetic disorder characterised by tumour formation within the nervous system with at least three distinct types. Type 2 tumours form within the central nervous system. Lisch nodules are characteristic of Type 1 neurofibromatosis.

34) e

Retinoblastoma is a tumour of immature retinal cells. It usually affects children under 5. The loss of the red reflex should prompt further examination in this age group and various treatments are available including enucleation of the eye.

35) h

Graves' disease is an autoimmune thyroid disease leading to hyperthyroidism. It is thought the same TSH receptor auto-antibodies which stimulate the thyroid bind to extraocular muscles leading to swelling behind the eye causing the appearance of bulging eyes.

36) b

Giant cell arteritis is as an inflammatory disorder of medium to large blood vessels; a common site for this to occur is the temporal artery. It is commonly associated with polymyalgia rheumatica. Cases are generally in those over 50 years old and require high-dose steroids if suspected to prevent blindness. The CRP levels and ESR will be raised.

37) a

Sudden loss of vision in a patient with a known ischaemic history should guide clinicians towards a vascular pathology for symptoms. The 'cherry red spot' appearance is due to the macula receiving blood from the posterior ciliary artery leading to a central perfused area whilst the surrounding retina is supplied via the retinal artery.

38)   f

Migraine is a visual disturbance with a headache in which there is often a family history. Patients may experience zig-zag lines, changes in vision and nausea which often recovers after several hours.

39)   d

Retinal detachment is a cause of sudden painless loss of vision. Symptoms include a sudden vision loss with floaters and flashes, and symptoms do not resolve. This is in comparison to migraine in which symptoms do resolve after several hours. Severe myopia is a risk factor for retinal detachment.

40)   h

Optic neuritis is inflammation of the optic nerve. Characteristic findings on fundoscopy are a swollen and pale optic disc. Uhthoff's phenomenon is the worsening of symptoms with an increase in body temperature and is another classical sign of MS.

41)   a

Open angle glaucoma is the most common form of glaucoma in the UK and is due to a gradual resistance to aqueous outflow. Symptoms are usually absent although ocular pressures are raised. It can be treated using beta-blockers to reduce aqueous secretion, carbonic anhydrase inhibitors to reduce aqueous secretion via the ciliary body, prostaglandin derivatives or alpha-2 stimulants which increase aqueous outflow via the uveoscleral route and muscarinic stimulants such as pilocarpine which increase ciliary muscle contraction to enhance aqueous outflow via the trabecular meshwork.

42) g

Cataracts are common in the elderly and can be age-related degenerative changes; in this case, they are known as senile cataracts. Patients may notice a gradual loss of clarity of vision. Other causes of cataracts include diabetes, Down's syndrome, myotonic dystrophy, corticosteroids and metabolic disorders such as Wilson's disease.

43) b

The macula is the central part of the retina and is responsible for central vision. The presence of an existing background diabetic retinopathy and changes in central vision should prompt investigations for a maculopathy. Treatment involves laser therapy or injections of anti-VEGF into the eye.

44) h

A bitemporal hemianopia is due to compression at the optic chiasm disrupting nasal fibres of both optic nerves. Causes include pituitary adenoma craniopharyngioma or an anterior communicating artery aneurysm.

45) e

Uncorrected refractive errors are common in children; however, a thorough history and examination should be performed to ensure that other symptoms are not missed to exclude cataracts and retinal disease such as retinitis pigmentosa.

Short answer question answers

1)

a. Acute closed angle glaucoma.   1 mark

b. Blockage of the trabecular meshwork by the iris at Schlemm's canal (1   2 marks
    mark), resulting in impairment of aqueous fluid drainage leading to an
    acute rise in intraocular pressure (1 mark).

c. Any 2 from: 2 marks
    - Hypermetropia.
    - Shallow anterior chamber.
    - Thicker lens.
    - Small corneal diameter.

d. Any 1 from: 3 marks
    - Supportive measures: analgesia, antiemetics.
    Any 2 from:
    - Acute drug: topical muscarinic stimulants, e.g. pilocarpine.
    - Systemic carbonic anhydrase inhibitors, e.g. acetazolamide.
    - Topical beta-blockers, e.g. timolol.
    - Sympathomimetics, e.g. apraclonidine.

e. Surgery or laser treatment to allow aqueous circulation when the   2 marks
    intraocular pressure is reduced (1 mark). Patients may need
    prophylactic surgery on the contralateral eye to prevent acute closed
    angle glaucoma (1 mark).

2)

a. Any 3 from: 3 marks
    - Episcleritis.
    - Scleritis.
    - Corneal foreign body or abrasion.
    - Ocular trauma.
    - Acute closed angle glaucoma.
    - Iritis.

- Subconjunctival haemorrhage.
- Anterior uveitis.
- Corneal ulcer.
- Keratitis.
- Corneal abscess.
- Blepharitis.
- Allergic or viral conjunctivitis.
- Endophthalmitis.

b. Any 2 from: 2 marks
- *Staphylococcus epidermidis.*
- *Staphylococcus aureus.*
- *Streptococcus pneumoniae.*
- *Haemophilus influenzae.*
- *Moraxella lacunata.*

c. Topical chloramphenicol.   2 marks
Any 2 from:
- Avoid touching eyes.
- Avoid sharing towels.
- Wash hands thoroughly after using eye drops.
- Return if condition persists.

d. Any 2 from: 1 mark
- Itchy eyes.
- Swelling.
- Watery discharge.
- Severe chemosis.

e. *Chlamydia trachomatis* — oral erythromycin for 2 weeks.   2 marks
Neisseria gonorrhoeae — single dose cefotaxime IM or 7 days IV
benzylpenicillin.

3)
a. Cataract.   1 mark
b. Any 3 from: 3 marks
- Increasing age.
- Excessive sunlight.

- Ionising radiation.
- Eye trauma.
- High myopia.
- Recurrent uveitis.
- Corticosteroid use.

c. Senile.   2 marks

Congenital.

d. Phacoemulsification.   1 mark

e. Endophthalmitis.   3 marks

Any 2 from:

- Intravitreal or intravenous antibiotics.
- Vitrectomy.
- Corticosteroids.

4)

a. Herpes zoster ophthalmicus.   2 marks

Varicella zoster virus.

b. A rash extending to the tip of the nose indicates nasociliary nerve   2 marks
involvement (1 mark) which increases the chance of ocular
complications (1 mark).

c. Ophthalmic division of the trigeminal nerve (V1).   1 mark

d. Patient: oral systemic antivirals, e.g. acyclovir, valaciclovir.   2 marks

Immunosuppressed patients: intravenous acyclovir.

e. Post-herpetic neuralgia.   3 marks

Any 2 from:

- Paracetamol.
- Codeine phosphate.
- Amitriptyline.
- Duloxetine.
- Gabapentin.
- Pregabalin.
- Topical capsaicin.

- Lidocaine plasters.
- Self-management advice including wearing loose clothing or protecting sensitive areas with a wound dressing.

5)

a.   Any 2 from: 2 marks
- Female gender.
- Granulomatosis with polyangiitis (Wegener's granulomatosis).
- Systemic lupus erythematosus (SLE).
- Polyarteritis nodosa.
- Vasculitis.
- Inflammatory bowel disease.
- Syphilis.
- Sarcoidosis.
- TB.
- Herpes zoster ophthalmicus.
- Trauma.
- Previous ocular surgery.

b.   Any 2 from: 2 marks
- Inflammation involves the full thickness of the sclera.
- Hyperaemia of superficial and deep episcleral vessels.
- Anterior uveitis.
- The whole circumference of the anterior segment affected.
- Scleral thinning.
- Corneal thinning.
- Perforation.

c.   Analgesia.   2 marks
Urgent ophthalmology referral.

d. ½ mark for each correct line from Table 10.1 below. 2 marks

Table 10.1

	Episcleritis	Scleritis
Incidence	Common	Uncommon
Onset	Fast	Gradual
Pain	Mild	Moderate to severe
Discharge	None	Watery
Inflammation	Superficial	All layers of sclera
Associated with systemic disease	Rare	Common
Visual disturbance	Rare	Common
Outcome	Settles itself within a week Can be recurrent	Can lead to blindness
Treatment	Self-limiting Topical NSAIDs	Topical steroids, Topical NSAIDs Immunosuppression

e. Any 2 from: 2 marks
- Supportive advice.
- Topical NSAIDs.
- Lubricating eye drops.

6)

a. Orbital cellulitis. 1 mark

b. Any 2 from: 2 marks
- *Streptococcus pneumoniae*.
- *Staphylococcus aureus*.

- *Streptococcus pyogenes.*
- *Haemophilus influenzae.*

c.   Any 2 from: 2 marks
- Ethmoidal sinusitis.
- Maxillary sinusitis.
- Pre-septal or facial infection.
- Dacryocystitis.
- Upper respiratory tract infection.
- Dental abscess.
- Septal perforation.
- Retained foreign body.
- Orbital surgery.
- Ocular surgery.
- Systemic infection in an immunocompromised individual.

d.   Hospital admission (1 mark) for IV broad-spectrum antibiotics (third-   2 marks
generation cephalosporins) (1 mark).

e.   Pre-septal cellulitis (1 mark) and ½ mark for each correct line from   3 marks
Table 10.2 below.

Table 10.2

	Orbital cellulitis	Pre-septal cellulitis
Visual acuity	May be reduced	Normal
Fever	Present	Present
Chemosis	Moderate	Absent or mild
Ocular mobility	Reduced	Normal
Pain on eye movement	Present	Absent
Colour vision	May be reduced	Normal
RAPD	Present	Absent
Proptosis	Present	None
Lid swelling	Severe	Mild-moderate

7)

a. Left (1 mark) sixth cranial nerve (1 mark).   2 marks

b. Supplies the lateral rectus muscle which is responsible for abduction   1 mark
of the eye for outward gaze.

c. Any 2 from: 2 marks
- Horizontal diplopia.
- Symptoms worse on distance vision.
- Increased diplopia when looking to the affected side.

d. Any 6 from: 3 marks
- Idiopathic.
- Microvascular ischaemia.
- Migraine headache.
- Neoplasms.
- Raised intracranial pressure.
- Giant cell arteritis.
- Basal skull fracture.
- Trauma.
- Multiple sclerosis.
- Sarcoidosis.
- Vasculitis.
- Meningitis.
- Cavernous sinus thrombosis.
- Carotid-cavernous fistula.
- Congenital.

e. Any 2 from: 2 marks
- Prisms.
- Occlusion.
- Botulinum toxin.

8)

a. Any 4 from: 2 marks
- Smoking.
- Hypertension.
- Obesity.

- Diabetes.
- Hyperlipidaemia.
- Aortic disease.
- Arrhythmias.
- Structural cardiac defects.
- Valvular heart disease.
- Endocarditis.
- Carotid artery disease.
- Antiphospholipid syndrome.
- Leukaemia.
- Lymphoma.
- Previous TIA or stroke.
- Renal disease.
- Thrombophilia.
- Vasculitis (giant cell arteritis, granulomatosis with polyangiitis, SLE, PAN, Kawasaki disease).
- Glaucoma.
- Syphilis.
- Lyme disease.
- Toxoplasmosis.
- Cocaine.
- Oral contraceptive pill.
- Trauma.
- Migraine.

b. Embolism.   1 mark

c. Any 2 from: 2 marks
  - RAPD.
  - Decreased visual acuity.
  - Visible emboli on fundoscopy.
  - Optic disc oedema.
  - Segmentation of blood in artery (cattle-trucking).
  - AF.
  - Carotid bruit.
  - Heart murmur.

d. Any 3 from: 3 marks
    ● CRP and ESR to exclude giant cell arteritis.
    ● Carotid ultrasound.
    ● ECG.
    ● Echo.
    ● Blood cultures.
    ● Clotting screen.
    ● Antiphospholipid screen.
    ● Vasculitis screen (ANA, ANCA, DNA, RF).
    ● Syphilis serology.

e. Any 2 from: 2 marks
    ● Branch occlusion — changes are limited to the retinal area supplied by the blood vessel.
    ● Branch occlusion — there may not be any symptoms if the area affected is away from the macula.
    ● Branch occlusion — there is no cherry red spot.

9)

a. Any 4 from: 2 marks
    ● Smoking.
    ● Obesity.
    ● Alcohol.
    ● High salt diet.
    ● Family history.
    ● Stress.
    ● Sedentary lifestyle.
    ● Hyperlipidaemia.

b. Any 4 from: 2 marks
    ● Generalised arteriolar narrowing.
    ● Arteriolar focal constriction.
    ● Exaggeration of the light reflex.
    ● Arteriovenous nipping (vein constriction).
    ● Cotton wool spots.

- Flame-shaped haemorrhages.
- Hard exudate.
- Retinal oedema.

c. 130/80mmHg.   1 mark

d. Any 2 from: 1 mark
- Central retinal artery occlusion.
- Branch retinal artery occlusion.
- Central retinal vein occlusion.
- Branch retinal vein occlusion.
- Macroaneurysms.
- Non-arteritic ischaemic optic neuropathy.
- Ocular motor nerve palsy.

e. Any 4 from: 4 marks
- ACE inhibitors.
- Calcium channel antagonists.
- Angiotensin II receptor antagonists.
- Thiazide diuretics.
- Beta-blockers.
- Alpha-blockers.
- Loop diuretics.
- Aldosterone antagonists.

10)
a. Pre-proliferative diabetic retinopathy.   2 marks
b. Any 3 from: 3 marks
- New blood vessel formation in proliferative disease.
- Macular oedema in diabetic maculopathy.
- Iris rubeosis.
- Vitreous haemorrhage.
- Retinal detachment.

c. Retinal vein occlusion.   2 marks
    Hypertensive retinopathy.

d.   Diabetic maculopathy.   1 mark

e.   Any 2 from: 2 marks

- Yearly diabetic retinal screening.
- Effective glucose control.
- Smoking cessation.
- Effective blood pressure control.
- Cholesterol reduction.
- Weight control.

11)

a.   Loss of central vision.   1 mark

b.   There are two types of ARMD — wet and dry (1 mark). The dry type   3 marks
is the presence of drusen and retinal pigment epithelial atrophy (1
mark). The wet type is the neovascularisation of the retina and
subsequent bleeding (1 mark).

c.   It is thought that drusen deposits within Bruch's membrane which   2 marks
separates retinal pigment epithelium and the retina from the
underlying choroidal blood supply leading to disruption of nutrient
delivery and removal causing retinal atrophy leading to dry ARMD (1
mark). Wet ARMD occurs if a break in Bruch's membrane occurs,
fragile blood vessels can grow directly into the retina and, if these are
damaged, haemorrhage and oedema results in loss of central vision
(1 mark).

d.   Any 4 from: 2 marks

- Increasing age.
- Family history.
- Smoking.
- Female gender.
- Obesity.
- Hypertension.
- Hypercholesterolaemia.
- Caucasian ethnicity.
- High exposure to sunlight.

e.   Any 4 from: 2 marks
   - Anti-VEGF therapy.
   - Photodynamic therapy.
   - Laser photocoagulation.
   - Counselling.
   - Amsler grid.
   - Smoking cessation.
   - High-dose antioxidants.
   - Registration as visually impaired.

12)

a.   Retinoblastoma.   1 mark

b.   Any 3 from: 3 marks
   - Cataract.
   - Vitreous maldevelopment.
   - Retinal dysplasia.
   - Corneal opacity.
   - Advanced retinopathy of prematurity.
   - Toxocara granuloma.

c.   Any 2 from: 2 marks
   - Ultrasound orbit.
   - CT head.
   - MRI head.
   - Genetic testing.

d.   Any 2 from: 2 marks
   - Laser therapy.
   - Cryotherapy.
   - Radiotherapy.
   - Chemotherapy.
   - Enucleation.

e.   Any 2 from: 2 marks
   - Prosthesis following enucleation.
   - Psychological counselling.

- Genetic counselling.
- Protective eye wear.
- Long-term follow-up and surveillance.

13)

a. The neurosensory layer containing photoreceptors and ganglion cells   1 mark
   and the retinal pigment epithelium.

b. Rhegmatogenous.   3 marks
   Tractional.
   Exudative.

c. Any 2 from: 2 marks
   - Retinal breaks.
   - Proliferative diabetic retinopathy.
   - Uveitis.
   - Intraocular tumours.
   - Central serous retinopathy.

d. Any 4 from: 2 marks
   - Floaters.
   - Flashing lights.
   - Loss of red reflex.
   - Distortion of straight lines.
   - RAPD.
   - Loss of central vision.

e. Any 2 from: 2 marks
   - Vitrectomy.
   - Scleral buckling.
   - Cryotherapy.
   - Laser photocoagulation.
   - Pneumatic retinopexy.

Chapter 11

Paediatrics
ANSWERS

Single best answers

1) b.
2) d.
3) a.
4) c.
5) a.
6) d.
7) c.
8) b.
9) c.
10) d.
11) c.
12) d.
13) a.
14) d.
15) d.
16) c.
17) a.
18) b.
19) b.
20) a.

21) a.
22) c.
23) a.

Extended matching question answers

1) f

   Turner syndrome (45XO) gives this appearance together with a short stature, obesity and fertility problems.

2) c

   Fragile X syndrome gives the features described and is the most common cause of sex-linked learning disability.

3) g

   Cri du chat syndrome gives a high-pitched 'cat-like' cry, but this cry is not pathognomonic of the condition.

4) a

   These are features of Down's syndrome; the iris speckles are Brushfield spots.

5) d

   Prader-Willi syndrome typically causes the mentioned features including hyperphagia.

6) c

   'Hyper' = over; tropia = manifest when both eyes are uncovered.

7) f

   'Exo' = outside; phoria = manifest when one eye is covered.

8) a

   'Eso' = inner.

9) h

'Hypo' = below.

10) d

'Hypo' = below.

11) b

Appendicitis may present insidiously rather than the typical central pain localising to the right iliac fossa.

12) h

Crying on the toilet and overflow diarrhoea (overflow) are key signs of constipation in a child.

13) c

These are typical features of intussusception.

14) g

Non-caseating epithelioid cell granulomata are found histologically in Crohn's disease and would not be found in the other diagnoses.

15) d

Painless haematuria is seen in a Meckel's diverticulum. The child has likely obstructed.

16) d

Scarlet fever involves a palpable 'sandpaper-like' rash leading to circumoral pallor.

17) h

Parvovirus B19 causes erythema infectiosum which is a rash spreading from the face but sparing the nose.

18) a

This is a classic presentation of chickenpox with a rash made up of the different stages of appearance; the rash can appear as a papule, vesicle, pustule or crust.

19) f

Crops of umbilicated papules are often caused by a molluscum infection.

20) c

Erythema multiforme starts on the extremities and spreads centrally.

21) e

This involves extrahepatic duct destruction leading to biliary obstruction, meaning there is a build-up of conjugated bilirubin.

22) a

This is a typical description of physiological jaundice, notably disappearing quickly and without intervention.

23) c

Galactosaemia is an inherited disorder of metabolism, presenting with developmental delay, jaundice and sepsis.

24) h

A G6PD deficiency can cause a haemolytic crisis by illness or drugs.

25) b

This is a Rhesus disease caused by Rhesus incompatibility due to a prior maternal sensitising event.

26) b

These are some of the features of hypothyroidism in children. The low-frequency cry is important here.

27) g

These are features of fetal alcohol syndrome. The criteria include typical facial abnormalities, intrauterine growth restriction and cranial and learning abnormalities.

28) a

Cystic fibrosis causes problems with the GI tract, respiratory system and liver or biliary systems.

29) h

Two typical features of phenylketonuria are pale blue eyes and an unusual musty or mousy odour.

30) e

In a patient with recurrent infections, neglect should be considered.

31) g

A VSD can cause a left sternal edge murmur.

32) h

An ASD can cause this murmur, and typically would not cause an acutely unwell child.

33) d

Most tetralogy of Fallot cases are now recognised antenatally or early in life. If not picked up early, tetralogy can cause cyanosis and dyspnoea. The pulmonary stenosis can cause a characteristic murmur, and tet spells and hypoxia on squatting after exercise.

34) c

Coarctation of the aorta, if severe, presents with severe cyanosis and dyspnoea in the first few weeks of life as the ductus arteriosus closes.

35) a

A patent ductus arteriosus will often cause a 'machinery' murmur.

36) c

Reflex anoxia can cause seizures, including those that present as generalised tonic clonic seizures.

37) h

The progressive seizures are typical of juvenile myoclonic epilepsy.

38) g

Dravet syndrome can have a variable presentation, but often involves severe myoclonic epilepsy in previously healthy infants. The onset is often <15 months.

39) b

This type of quick recovery is typical of syncope. There may still be a few jerking movements without significant seizures.

40) f

This is characteristic of an absence seizure.

41) b

AML is more typical in adulthood. Certain congenital diseases such as Down's syndrome increases the likelihood of this disease in childhood.

42) f

A Wilms' tumour is the most common renal malignancy in childhood, and usually presents by the age of 5.

43) a

The t(9;22)(q34.1;q11.2) or Philadelphia chromosome is associated with ALL but is more commonly seen in chronic myeloid leukaemia.

44)   c

Ewing sarcoma has an onion-skin appearance on X-ray and presents with a mass that can be painful.

45)   d

Reed-Sternberg cells occur in Hodgkin's lymphoma.

Short answer question answers

1)

a. Right ventricular outflow tract obstruction.   4 marks
   Ventricular septal defect.
   Overriding aorta.
   Right ventricular hypertrophy.

b. Any 2 from: 2 marks
   - Systolic thrill at the lower left sternal border.
   - Aortic ejection click.
   - Loud systolic murmur in the pulmonary area.
   - Ejection systolic murmur.

c. Any 2 from: 2 marks
   - Low oxygen saturations.
   - Cyanosis.
   - Low birthweight.
   - Poor growth.
   - Poor feeding.
   - Shortness of breath.
   - Squatting.
   - Tet spells.

d. Right axis deviation.   1 mark

e. Atrial septal defect.   1 mark

2)

a. Any 3 from: 3 marks
   - Sickle cell disease.
   - Cystic fibrosis.
   - Congenital hypothyroidism.
   - Phenylketonuria (PKU).
   - Maple syrup urine disease (MSUD).

- Medium-chain acyl-CoA dehydrogenase deficiency.
- Isovaleric acidaemia.
- Glutaric aciduria Type 1.
- Homocystinuria.

b. Any 2 from: 2 marks
- Congenital cataracts.
- Congenital heart disease.
- Undescended testes.
- Developmental dysplasia of the hip.
- Newborn hearing screening.

c. Any 2 from: 2 marks
- Pale blue eyes.
- Musty or mousy colour.
- Developmental delay.
- Learning disability.
- Vomiting.
- Skin eczema.
- Scleroderma-like lesions.
- Seizures.
- Behavioural disturbance.

d. Any 2 from: 2 marks
- Feeding difficulties.
- Lethargy.
- Low-frequency cry.
- Hoarse cry.
- Constipation.
- Large fontanelles.
- Goitre.
- Myxoedema.
- Pericardial effusion.
- Macroglossia.
- Bradycardia.
- Cardiomegaly.

- Hypotonia.
- Jaundice.
- Hypothermia.

e. PKU is due to a phenylalanine hydroxylase deficiency (0.5 marks), **1 mark**
    leading to a build-up of phenylpyruvic acid and phenylethylamine; the
    byproducts are neurotoxic (0.5 marks).

3)

a. Barlow test — gentle backward pressure applied to the head of each **4 marks**
    femur to palpably displace the hip.
    Ortolani test — gentle forward pressure applied to the head of each
    femur to reduce posteriorly displaced femoral head.

b. Ultrasound.   **1 mark**

c. Any 1 from: **1 mark**
    - Reduced alpha and beta angles.
    - Reduced bony coverage of the femoral epiphysis.

d. Any 2 from: **2 marks**
    - Premature joint degeneration.
    - Arthritis.
    - Chronic lower back pain.
    - Delay in walking.
    - Avascular necrosis.

e. Any 2 from: **2 marks**
    - Bracing.
    - Flexion-abduction orthosis/Pavlik harness.
    - Surgery.

4)

a. Any 3 from: **3 marks**
    - Abnormal fidgeting.
    - Asymmetry.
    - Hypotonia.
    - Spasticity.

- Dystonia.
- Abnormal motor development.

b. Neonatal encephalopathy.   1 mark

c. Spastic.   3 marks
   Athetoid.
   Ataxic.

d. APGAR   1 mark

e. Any 2 from: 2 marks
   - Diazepam.
   - Baclofen.
   - Trihexyphenidyl.
   - Levodopa.
   - Botulinum toxin type A.

5)

a. Any 2 from: 2 marks
   - Recurrent regurgitation.
   - Vomiting.
   - Failure to thrive.
   - Cough.
   - Feeding problems.
   - Wheeze.
   - Choking.

b. Any 2 from: 2 marks
   - Obesity.
   - Prematurity.
   - Hiatus hernia.
   - Family history.
   - Congenital diaphragmatic hernia.
   - Oesophageal atresia.

c. Any 2 from: 1 mark
   - Endoscopy.
   - 24-hour oesophageal pH.

- Manometry.
- Barium meal.

d. Vomiting — forceful and active.   1 mark
   Reflux — sphincter incompetence.

e. Any 4 from: 4 marks
   - Lethargy.
   - Irritability.
   - Altered mental state.
   - Bulging fontanelle.
   - Pyrexia.
   - Abdominal distention/mass.
   - Bile-stained vomit.
   - Rapidly increasing head size.
   - Chronic diarrhoea.
   - Blood in stool.
   - Haematemesis.
   - Forceful vomiting.

6)

a. Any 3 from: 3 marks
   - Age of onset 2-8 weeks.
   - Non-bilious vomiting.
   - Projectile vomiting.
   - Occurs 30-60 minutes after feeding.
   - Increasing over a short period of time.
   - Increasing in intensity.

b. 'Olive'-mass (1 mark), best felt in the epigastrium (1 mark).   2 marks

c. Ultrasound.   1 mark

d. Correct the electrolyte abnormality.   2 marks
   Pyloromyotomy.

e. Hypochloraemia.   2 marks
   Hypokalaemia.
   Metabolic alkalosis.

7)

a. Any 4 from: 2 marks

- Normal colour of skin, lips and tongue.
- Responds normally to social cues.
- Content and smiles.
- Stays awake or wakens quickly.
- Strong normal cry.
- Normal skin turgor.

b. Any 4 from: 2 marks

- Pallor.
- Does not respond normally to social cues.
- Does not smile.
- Wakes only with prolonged stimulation.
- Decreased activity.
- Nasal flaring.
- Tachypnoea.
- Oxygen saturations ≤95% in air.
- Crackles.
- Poor feeding.
- Dry mucous membranes.
- Capillary refill time ≥3 seconds.
- Reduced urine output.
- Tachycardia.
- Temperature ≥39°C (3-6 months of age).
- Rigors.
- Fever ≥5 days.
- Swelling of a limb or joint.
- Not able to put weight on limb.

c. Any 4 from: 2 marks

- Appears ill.
- Pale or mottled.
- Ashen or blue.
- No response to social cues.
- Unable to rouse.

- Weak or high-pitched cry.
- Grunting.
- Tachypnoea >60 breaths per minute.
- Moderate or severe chest indrawing.
- Reduced skin turgor.
- Temperature ≥38°C (0-3 months of age).
- Non-blanching rash.
- Bulging fontanelle.
- Neck stiffness.
- Status epilepticus.
- Focal neurological signs.
- Focal seizures.

d. All green features — give advice.   3 marks

Any amber features — information on warning symptoms, specified follow-up, ensure direct access.

Any red features — urgent assessment by a paediatric specialist.

e. Give oxygen to keep saturations above 94%.   1 mark

Take at least one set of blood cultures.

Give broad-spectrum IV antibiotics.

Give IV fluids.

Measure lactate.

Measure urine output.

8)

a. An inflammatory condition where bronchial hyper-responsiveness   2 marks
(0.5 marks) leads to paroxysmal (0.5 marks), reversible (0.5 marks) airway obstruction (0.5 marks).

b. Any 3 from: 3 marks
- PEFR <33% of best/predicted.
- Oxygen saturations <92%.
- Silent chest.
- Cyanosis.
- Poor respiratory effort.

- Arrhythmia.
- Hypotension.
- Exhaustion.
- Altered consciousness.

c. Inhaled daily steroid. 1 mark

d. Oxygen. 3 marks

Salbutamol and ipratropium nebulised in oxygen.

Prednisolone or hydrocortisone.

e. Severe asthma that does not respond well to intermediate care. 1 mark

9)

a. At least two unprovoked seizures (1 mark) >24 hours apart (1 mark). 2 marks

b. A seizure is the transient occurrence of signs or symptoms (1 mark) 2 marks
due to abnormal electrical activity in the brain (1 mark).

c. Focal (0.5 marks) and generalised (0.5 marks). 1 mark

d. SUDEP — sudden unexpected death in epilepsy (1 mark); a sudden, 3 marks
unexpected, unwitnessed, non-traumatic, non-drowning death of a
person with epilepsy (1 mark), in whom postmortem examination
does not reveal a structural or toxicological cause of death (1 mark).

e. Any 2 from: 2 marks

- Migraine.
- Parasomnias.
- Syncope.
- Cardiac arrhythmia.
- Non-epileptic attack.
- Panic attack.
- Hyperventilation.
- Drop attack.
- TIA.
- Paroxysmal vertigo.
- Hypoglycaemia.
- Encephalopathy.

10)

a. Oligoarticular juvenile idiopathic arthritis.   2 marks

b. Positive antinuclear antibodies (ANA).   1 mark

c. Any 2 from: 2 marks
    - Eyes (uveitis).
    - Nails/skin (rashes, psoriasis, dactylitis, pitting).
    - Tendons/ligaments (enthesitis).
    - Hepatosplenomegaly.
    - Pericardial effusions.

d. Any 3 from: 3 marks
    - NSAIDs.
    - Steroids.
    - Methotrexate.
    - Sulfasalazine.
    - Leflunomide.
    - Etanercept.
    - Tocilizumab.

e. Any 2 from: 2 marks
    - Fever >39°C.
    - Typical rash.
    - Transient erythema.
    - Pharyngitis.
    - Leucocytosis >80% polymorphs.
    - Glycosylated ferritin <20%.

11)

a. AML is the malignant transformation of myeloid progenitor cells.   2 marks
    ALL is the malignant transformation of lymphoid progenitor cells.

b. Any 4 from: 2 marks
    - Fatigue.
    - Malaise.
    - Joint pain.
    - Recurrent infections.

- Fever.
- Splenomegaly.
- Dyspnoea.
- Headache.
- Features of meningism.
- Bleeding.
- Bruising.
- Cranial nerve palsies.
- Pallor.
- Petechiae.
- Lymphadenopathy.
- Abdominal distention.
- Gum hypertrophy.

c. Any 1 from: 1 mark
- Blast cells.
- Reduced number of mature cells.

d. Any 3 from: 3 marks
- Chemotherapy.
- Transfusion.
- Corticosteroids.
- Methotrexate.
- Stem-cell transplantation.
- Growth factors.
- Allopurinol.

e. Any 2 from: 2 marks
- Haemorrhage.
- Infection.
- Anaemia.
- Graft vs. host disease.
- Hair loss.
- Skin changes.
- Tumour lysis syndrome.
- Electrolyte disturbances.

- Liver and kidney toxicity.
- Peripheral neuropathy.
- Infertility.
- Cardiomyopathy.
- Lung fibrosis.
- Hypothyroidism.
- Growth delay.
- Death.

12)

a. Emotional.   2 marks
   Physical.
   Sexual.
   Neglect.

b. Any 3 from: 3 marks
- Previous history of abuse.
- Mental/physical health issue.
- Disability in the carer.
- Financial problems.
- Single parent.
- Children in care.
- Domestic violence.
- Drug/alcohol misuse in carers.
- Disability or chronic illness in child.
- History of animal mistreatment.

c. Any 2 from: 2 marks
- Communication from other agencies.
- Presence of risk factors.
- Findings on history/examination.
- Observation during consultation.
- Disclosure by child/carer.

d. Any 2 from: 2 marks
- Fractures of different ages.
- Explanation not consistent with injury.

- Occult fractures on X-ray.
- Child not mobile.

e. Any 1 from: 1 mark
- Child protection leads in the trust.
- Police.
- Social workers.
- NSPCC.
- Local safeguarding board.
- Government websites.

13)

a. Any 2 from: 2 marks
- *Haemophilus influenzae* B.
- *Neisseria meningitidis*.
- *Streptococcus pneumoniae*.
- *Listeria monocytogenes*.
- *Escherichia coli*.

b. Any 3 from: 3 marks
- Fever.
- Neck stiffness.
- Headache.
- Photophobia.
- Back rigidity.
- Altered mental state.
- Shock.
- Kernig's sign.
- Brudzinski's sign.
- Focal neurological deficit.
- Seizures.

c. Haemorrhagic (petechial/purpuric). 2 marks
Non-blanching.

d. Lumbar puncture. 1 mark

e.   Any 2 from: 2 marks

- IV ceftriaxone.
- Dexamethasone.
- Vancomycin if recent foreign travel.
- Corticosteroids.
- Analgesia.
- Antipyretic.

Chapter 12

Psychiatry
ANSWERS

Single best answers

1) a.
2) b.
3) b.
4) d.
5) d.
6) c.
7) a.
8) c.
9) c.
10) c.
11) d.
12) a.
13) d.
14) b.
15) c.
16) d.
17) c.
18) b.
19) d.
20) c.

21) b.
22) d.
23) b.

Extended matching question answers

1) f

An emotionally unstable personality disorder is characterised by fears of abandonment, impulsivity and outbursts of emotion which can result in suicidal thoughts. Emotionally unstable personality disorder is often used interchangeably with 'borderline' personality disorder.

2) a

A paranoid personality disorder is characterised by suspiciousness and feelings of betrayal particularly around perceived infidelity of their spouse or sexual partner.

3) c

A histrionic personality disorder may present with the continuous seeking of approval, flirtation or provocative behaviour and the desire to be the centre of attention.

4) b

Patients with a dissocial (antisocial) personality disorder behave dangerously and sometimes illegally; they tend to behave aggressively and may have a criminal record.

5) g

An anankastic personality disorder is also known as obsessional or obsessive-compulsive personality disorder. Patients are perfectionist with rigid, inflexible regimes and set unrealistically high standards.

6) b

Risperidone is an example of an atypical antipsychotic. Other examples include quetiapine, olanzapine and aripiprazole. Typical antipsychotics include haloperidol and flupentixol.

7)   d

Venlafaxine and duloxetine are selective serotonin-norepinephrine reuptake inhibitors (SNRI).

8)   a

Trazadone is a serotonin antagonist and reuptake inhibitor (SARI).

9)   c

Lithium is a mood stabiliser which is not a mechanism but the effect of the drug. Several different anticonvulsant medications can be used as mood stabilizers, e.g. valproate.

10)   h

Lorazepam is an example of a benzodiazepine. Most benzodiazepines end in the suffix –pam; chlordiazepoxide is an exception to this.

11)   e

Hypochondriacal disorder is the persistent preoccupation with having a physical health disorder. Normal sensations are perceived as abnormal and evidence of a health condition.

12)   f

Somatisation disorder is characterised by multiple and recurrent physical health (somatic) symptoms that cannot be explained by a medical condition.

13)   h

Malingering is not strictly a medical diagnosis and is the fabrication of mental or physical symptoms for personal gain such as financial reward or avoiding work.

14)   b

Dissociative amnesia is a retrograde loss of memory not due to an organic mental disorder in the absence of anterograde amnesia. This is centred around a traumatic event and resolves within a short time. A dissociative fugue has all the features of dissociative amnesia but involves unexpected, purposeful travel away from home.

15) g

Dissociative convulsions are also known as non-epileptic seizures.

16) f

Creutzfeldt-Jakob disease is a rare, fatal cause of dementia caused by misfiled proteins called prions.

17) a

Alzheimer's disease is the most common cause of dementia and is thought to be a build-up of amyloid plaques and tau protein.

18) h

Huntington's disease is an autosomal dominant disorder caused by expansion of the CAG triple in the Huntingtin gene.

19) d

Normal pressure hydrocephalus (NPH) presents with a triad of gait disturbance, dementia and urinary incontinence. NPH is the only cause of dementia listed in the question that is potentially fully reversible.

20) e

Vascular dementia is caused by issues with the supply of blood to the brain, leading to a progressive cognitive decline that occurs in a stepwise manner. Differentiating dementia syndromes can be challenging, due to the frequently overlapping clinical features and related underlying pathology.

21) g

Cognitive behavioural therapy (CBT) is a talking therapy that aims to manage problems by modifying thinking and behaviours. It is based on cycles of thinking and actions, and deals with current problems rather than past issues. Dialectical behavioural therapy is a talking therapy based on CBT that has been modified to help service users with intense emotions such as with a borderline personality disorder.

22) c

Sensate focus therapy is a couple's therapy aiming to build trust and intimacy, and create a more satisfying sexual relationship using stages of touching and feedback.

23) f

Eye movement desensitisation therapy was developed as a trauma-based therapy, often used in post-traumatic stress disorder. The client is asked to recall distressing memories and then whilst generating lateral eye movements or hand tapping.

24) a

Flooding is a form of exposure therapy where patients are directly exposed to their phobias for an extended period of time in a safe and controlled environment. Systematic desensitisation is also known as graded exposure therapy; the patient is gradually exposed to the phobic stimulus until it can be tolerated.

25) h

Interpersonal therapy focuses on relationships and how psychological symptoms are a response to difficulties in everyday interactions with other people. Family therapy encompasses a range of different therapies which, as the name suggests, involves the family. It has a wide variety of uses including in child and adolescent mental health and behavioural problems, and includes discussion around support, behaviour, interactions and problem solving.

26) b

Othello syndrome is also known as pathological jealousy and morbid jealousy. A person with Othello syndrome has delusions that their partner is being unfaithful without evidence to support this with inappropriate behaviour such as repeated interrogation and stalking.

27) g

De Clerambault's syndrome, also known as erotomania, is characterised by a delusion typically in a young female that a male of higher social standing is in love with her. There has been little to no contact between the two prior to the delusion and it has not been encouraged by the victim.

28) d

Ekbom's syndrome, also known as delusional parasitosis, is a delusional disorder in which the patient believes that they are infested with parasites or insects. They typically report formication which is a form of tactile hallucinations.

29) f

Capgras syndrome is the belief that a friend, partner or family member has been replaced by an identical imposter; it is also known as imposter syndrome.

30) a

Cotard syndrome is a rare disorder in which the affected person holds the delusional belief that they are dead, do not exist, are putrefying, or have lost their blood or internal organs.

31) c

Acamprosate is used to maintain abstinence from alcohol and reduce cravings.

32) f

Buprenorphine has partial opioid agonist and opioid antagonist activity. It is used for opioid drug dependence as a sublingual tablet. The high affinity for opioid receptors reduces the impact of other opioids by preventing them from receptor binding. The patch form is used in the management of chronic pain.

33) e

Varenicline is a selective nicotine-receptor partial agonist used to treat nicotine addiction and reduces cravings and withdrawal symptoms.

34) b

Disulfiram is also known as Antabuse. It is used in alcohol dependence and causes the patient to feel unwell if they consume alcohol by inhibiting acetaldehyde dehydrogenase which leads to acetaldehyde build-up and unpleasant symptoms.

35) a

Methadone is typically green in colour and is used for the treatment of opioid dependency often as a heroin substitute.

36) f

Thought broadcasting is the belief that others can hear or read an individual's thoughts. This is different to thought echo in which the individual hears their thoughts spoken out loud.

37) b

Somatic passivity is the belief or feeling that the individual is a passive recipient of thoughts, sensations and actions from external forces.

38) c

Thought insertion is the feeling that thoughts have been pushed into the individual's mind and are not their own.

39) d

Delusional perception describes a false meaning attached to a normal event as described in the example.

40) e

Third person auditory hallucinations occur in the form of a running commentary or describing intended actions in the third person.

41) d

Neologisms are formations of new words.

42) c

Clanging also known as clang-associated is speech which is related by sounds rather than meaning, e.g. "I was in the street and saw a dog, frog, log, the woods, should".

43) e

Word salad, also known as incoherence, is unintelligible speech due to a mixture of random words and phrases.

44) g

Pressured speech is difficult to interrupt and can present in several different mental health conditions, but typically in bipolar affective disorder during a manic or hypomanic episode.

45) b

Perseveration is repetition of a word of phrase, for example, answering "yes" repeatedly to different questions. Perseveration can occur with behaviours.

Short answer question answers

1)

a. Any 3 from: 3 marks
- Paranoid delusions.
- Delusional perceptions.
- Thought broadcasting.
- Self-neglect.
- Auditory hallucinations.

b. Any 2 from: 2 marks
- Paranoid.
- Hebephrenic.
- Catatonic.
- Undifferentiated.
- Residual.
- Simple.

c. Any 2 from: 2 marks
- Chlorpromazine.
- Flupentixol.
- Fluphenazine.
- Haloperidol.
- Prochlorperazine.
- Zuclopenthixol.

d. Any 4 from: 2 marks
- Acute dystonic reaction.
- Akathisia.
- Parkinsonism.
- Tardive dyskinesia.

e. Clozapine.   1 mark

2)

a. Bipolar I features depression and episodes of mania. Patients with   1 mark
    bipolar I disorder may only have manic episodes whilst in bipolar II,
    depression is the more prominent feature, with episodes of
    hypomania.

b. Any 1 from each category: 4 marks
    i.   behaviour: excitable, over-friendly, inappropriate, agitation;
    ii. speech: pressured, fast, difficult to interrupt;
    iii. mood: elated, irritable;
    iv. thoughts: flight of ideas, clanging, tangentiality, grandiosity,
    circumstantiality.

c. Atypical antipsychotic.   1 mark

d. Any 2 from: 2 marks
    - Sodium valproate.
    - Carbamazepine.
    - Lamotrigine.

e. Any 2 from: 2 marks
    - Self-neglect.
    - Self-harm.
    - Financial vulnerability.
    - Sexual disinhibition.
    - Aggression.

3)

a. Low mood.   3 marks
    Anhedonia.
    Anergia.

b. Any 4 from: 4 marks
    - Full blood count: anaemia, infection, chronic inflammation.
    - Haematinics: iron, B12, folate deficiency.
    - Thyroid function tests: thyroid disorders.
    - Liver function tests: hepatic impairment, alcohol excess.
    - U&E: electrolyte imbalance, uraemia, CKD, dehydration.

- Blood glucose: diabetes.
- Vitamin D: vitamin D deficiency.
- Calcium profile: hypercalcaemia associated with mood changes.

c. Any 1 from: 1 mark
- Patient Health Questionnaire (PHQ-9).
- Hospital Anxiety and Depression Scale (HADS).
- Beck Depression Inventory (BDI).

d. Any 1 from: 1 mark
- Citalopram.
- Escitalopram.
- Fluoxetine.
- Fluvoxamine.
- Paroxetine.
- Sertraline.

e. Any 1 from: 1 mark
- Abdominal pain.
- Constipation.
- Diarrhoea.
- Nausea.
- Vomiting.

4)

a. Any 2 from: 2 marks
- Denial.
- Anger.
- Bargaining.
- Depression.
- Acceptance.

b. An abnormal perception in the absence of an external stimulus.   2 marks

c. Illusion.   1 mark

d. Any 4 from: 4 marks
- Cause of death unknown.
- Deceased not seen by certifying doctor either after death or within 14 days before death.

- Death was violent, unnatural or suspicious.
- Death may be due to an accident.
- Death due to self-neglect or neglect by others.
- Death may be due to industrial disease or related to employment.
- Death during operation or before recovery from effects of anaesthesia.
- Death occurring during or shortly after detention in police or prison custody.

e. Prolonged grief reaction.   1 mark

5)
a. Any 4 from: 2 marks
- Paracetamol.
- FBC.
- U&E.
- Bicarbonate.
- VBG.
- LFTs.
- Clotting.

b. N-acetylcysteine.   1 mark

c. Any 4 from: 4 marks
- Intent of overdose.
- Previous attempts.
- Planned.
- Previous psychiatric history.
- Alcohol use.
- Illicit substances.
- Past medical history.
- Significant life events.
- Social support.
- Ongoing suicidal ideation.
- Feelings about attempt.

- Final acts.
- Contacted help.
- Protective factors.

d. Any 2 from: 2 marks
  - Friends.
  - Family.
  - Primary care doctor.
  - Support line.
  - Emergency department.
  - Crisis helpline.

e. A Mental Health Act Assessment.   1 mark

6)

a. Any 3 from: 3 marks
  - Pyrexia.
  - Muscle rigidity.
  - Altered mental state.
  - Tachycardia.
  - Sweating.
  - Labile blood pressure.
  - Tremor.

b. Any 2 from: 2 marks
  - Use of neuroleptic medication.
  - Withdrawal of anti-parkinsonian medication.
  - High-dose medication.
  - Depot medication.
  - Agitation.
  - Previous episode of NMS.
  - Genetic predisposition.

c. Dopamine D2 receptor.   2 marks
   Dopamine.

d. Any 2 from: 2 marks
  - Stop antipsychotic medication.
  - IV fluids.

- Antipyretic medication.
- Cooling devices, e.g. fans.
- Muscle relaxants (includes dantrolene and bromocriptine).

e.   Benzodiazepines.   1 mark

7)

a.   The Deprivation of Liberty Safeguards.   1 mark

b.   Any 2 from: 2 marks
- Assume capacity unless established otherwise.
- Decisions must be made in the best interests of the patient.
- Help can be provided to make a decision for themselves (all practicable steps).
- People with capacity have the right to make an unwise decision.
- Decisions made for other people should be the least restrictive option.

c.   Can the patient understand (1 mark), retain (1 mark), weigh (1 mark)   4 marks
and communicate (1 mark)?

d.   Independent Mental Capacity Advocate.   1 mark

e.   A legally binding decision (1 mark) allowing someone whilst still   2 marks
capable, to state treatments that they do not want should they in the
future lack capacity to make this decision (1 mark).

8)

a.   Any 8 from: 4 marks
- Sweating.
- Clenched fists.
- Clenched teeth.
- Shaking.
- Staring.
- Restlessness.
- Change in tone of voice.
- Avoiding eye contact.
- Muscle tension.

- Change in breathing pattern.
- Loud speech.
- Abusive language.
- Banging.
- Kicking.
- Verbal threats.
- Flushed or pale face.
- Pacing.
- Gesturing.

b. Lorazepam or haloperidol.   2 marks
   Oral.

c. Procyclidine.   1 mark

d. Any 1 from: 1 mark
   - Torsade des pointes.
   - Ventricular arrhythmia.
   - Sudden death.

e. Any 2 from: 2 marks
   - Congenital long QT.
   - Medication.
   - Electrolyte imbalance (hypokalaemia, hypomagnesaemia, hypocalcaemia).
   - Hypothermia.
   - Cardiac disease.

9)

a. Any 4 from: 4 marks
   - Chest pain.
   - Palpitations.
   - Sweating.
   - Dry mouth.
   - Shortness of breath.
   - Nausea.
   - Dizziness.

- Sensory disturbance.
- Derealisation.

b. Panic disorder is regular, sudden or unexpected attacks of panic or 1 mark
    fear (panic attacks).

c. Any 2 from: 2 marks
    - Beck Anxiety Inventory (BAI).
    - General Health Questionnaire.
    - Hamilton Anxiety Scale.
    - Hospital Anxiety and Depression Scale (HADS).

d. Any 2 from: 2 marks
    - Patient education.
    - Self-help.
    - Relaxation therapy.
    - Cognitive behavioural therapy (CBT).

e. Selective serotonin-noradrenaline reuptake inhibitor/SNRI.   1 mark

10)

a. Units = strength (ABV as percentage) x volume (ml)/1000.   1 mark
    Daily units = 8 x 3000/1000 = 24.
    Weekly units = 24 x 7 = 168 units.

b. C — Have people ever told you to cut down your alcohol intake?   2 marks
    A — Have you been annoyed by people criticising your drinking?
    G — Have you ever felt guilty about your drinking?
    E — Do you need an eye-opener in the mornings?

c. Any 4 from: 4 marks
    - Withdrawal symptoms upon stopping.
    - Craving.
    - Tolerance.
    - Preoccupation with alcohol.
    - Continued drinking despite harmful consequences.
    - Primacy.
    - Narrowing of repertoire.

d. Reducing regime: chlordiazepoxide or lorazepam. 2 marks
Supplement: Pabrinex® or vitamin B compound or thiamine.

e. Any 1 from: 1 mark
- Acamprosate.
- Naltrexone.

11)

a. BMI = Weight (kg)/Height^2 (m) = 17.1 (1) kg/m^2. 2 marks

b. Any 4 from: 4 marks
- Bradycardia.
- Cold hands/feet.
- Thinning of hair.
- Lanugo hair.
- Dry skin.
- Ankle oedema.
- Evidence of self-harm.
- Acid erosion.
- Callus on back of hands.
- Hypotension.
- Hypothermia.

c. Any 2 from: 2 marks
- Dread of fatness.
- Distorted body image.
- Weight loss measures, e.g. extreme dieting.
- Laxative abuse.
- Restricted dietary choice.
- Amenorrhoea.

d. Any 1 from: 1 mark
- Family therapy.
- Cognitive behavioural therapy.

e. Refeeding syndrome. 1 mark

12)

a. Any 6 from: 3 marks

- FBC.
- U&E.
- LFTs.
- TFTs.
- FSH.
- LH.
- Oestradiol.
- Testosterone.
- Glucose.

b. Any 2 from: 2 marks

- Amenorrhoea.
- Oligomenorrhoea.
- Galactorrhoea.
- Breast tenderness.
- Breast pain.
- Vaginal dryness.

c. Any 2 from: 2 marks

- Citalopram.
- Escitalopram.
- Fluvoxamine.
- Paroxetine.
- Sertraline.

d. Any 2 from: 2 marks

- Pregnancy.
- Breastfeeding.
- Stress.
- Pituitary tumour.
- Prolactinoma.
- Post-ictal.
- Hypothyroidism.
- Liver cirrhosis.

e.   Any 1 from: 1 mark
  - Antipsychotics.
  - Tricyclic antidepressants.

13)

a.   Any 1 from: 1 mark
  - Police station.
  - Psychiatric hospital.
  - Emergency department.
  - Home.
  - Family.
  - Friend's home.

b.   Section 5(4).   1 mark

c.   i. Detention for assessment.   2 marks
     ii. 28 days.

d.   Any 4 from: 4 marks
  - Psychiatrist.
  - Psychologist.
  - Psychiatric nurse.
  - Occupational therapist.
  - Social worker.
  - Physiotherapist.
  - Pharmacist.
  - Approved mental health professional.
  - Key worker/care coordinator.

e.   The service user has to meet certain supervised conditions in the   2 marks
     community (1 mark); if they do not meet the conditions in the
     community treatment order such as complying with medication, they
     can be recalled to hospital (1 mark).